INTERMITTENT FASTING DIET FOR WOMEN OVER 50

A COMPLETE GUIDE TO IMPROVE YOUR EATING HABITS WITH HEALTHY AND CLEAN MEALS AND LOSE WEIGHT. HIGH PROTEIN RECIPES AND PLAN DIET FOR ATHLETES

Table of Contents

Introduction

Without a doubt, our bodies and our metabolic rate change when we reach menopause. One of the most important changes experienced by women over 50 is that they have a slower metabolic process and begin to gain weight. Fasting can be an unusual way to avoid this weight and also change the gain.

The studies try to show that this model fasting helps control hunger, and people who do not regularly even experience the same aspirations of others. If you are over 50 years old and also try to slow down the metabolic process, recurring fasting can help you stop consuming too much daily. Your body also begins to establish some chronic conditions such as high cholesterol and hypertension when it reaches 50 years. Intermittent fasting has been exposed to reduce cholesterol and blood stress, even without a fantastic offer of weight reduction. If you began to see your numbers improve every year in the doctor's work environment, you might have the opportunity to reduce them on an empty stomach, even without losing much weight. Recurring fasting may not be an exceptional idea for all single women. Anyone with a specific health condition or who often tends to be hypoglycemic should talk to a doctor. This new dietary pattern has special benefits for women who naturally store more fat in their bodies and may also have difficulty getting rid of these fat deposits.

Because women need intermittent fasting for women

For those interested in losing weight, intermittent fasting may seem like an excellent option. However, many people would like to know if women should fast. Is intermittent fasting reliable for women? There have been a couple of studies of study essential for the intermittent fasting can help you lose weight in this fascinating new food trend. Intermittent fasting is also called alternative daily fasting, although there are some variations in this diet plan. The American Journal of Clinical Nutrition recently conducted a research study that included 16 overweight men and women in a 10-week program. On fasting days, people absorbed food up to 25% of their approximate energy needs. The rest of the time, they received dietary training; however, they were not given a particular criterion to meet during this period. What made this exploration fascinating is that many people need to lose even more weight than those who study the research before seeing the same settings. It was a fantastic discovery that encouraged a large number of people to try fasting. Intermittent fasting for women has some positive results. Women with a healthy diet and training strategy may have problems with persistent fat; however, fasting is a reasonable solution for this.

Effects of intermittent fasting on weight loss

The desire to eat is the uncontrolled desire to eat caused by external forces; this occurs in times of war and shortage when food is limited. Food is easily served, but we choose not to eat it due to health and spiritual well-being or for other reasons. Fasting is as old as humanity, long before any other type of diet. Older people, like the Greeks, recognized that there was something naturally sensitive to routine fasting. Before the introduction of agriculture, people never ate 3 dishes a day plus intermediate snacks. When we find foods that can be separate days or human resources, we take them alone. From a development perspective, taking 3 meals a day is not a necessity to survive. Otherwise, we really shouldn't have endured it.

Fasting is inappropriate for service! Food manufacturers advise us to eat many dishes and take care of even one day. Fasting has no main period. It can be done from a few hours to several days or months. Recurring fasting is a food model in which one passes from one fast to another. Fasting has been involved by millions and countless people for countless years. Numerous studies have revealed that it has enormous benefits for well-being.

How IF affects women at this age and how to handle them

As health, diet, reproducibility, and nutritional needs change for mature and menopausal women, their relationships with intermittent fasting can be very different from those of young women. For example, while young women should pay attention to how intermittent fasting can affect their fertility levels, older women can freely practice intermittent fasting without these concerns. Therefore, older women can apply intermittent fasting weight loss techniques to their own lives (and lives) without worrying about the negative side effect that may arise in the future. However, for menopausal women, the situation is slightly different from that of fully mature women. People who go through menopause are dealing with daily hormonal fluctuations that cause hot flashes, insomnia, anxiety, irregular periods, and more. At the beginning of this process, intermittent fasting will not necessarily help and may even make your situation more stressful. For women in this situation who are actively going through menopause, they should remember that their body is extremely sensitive to changes at this time. If you find that intermittent fasting helps and that short periods of fasting are effective, you should also make sure to increase the intensity of fasting as gradually as possible so that your body can adapt without creating horrible hormonal repercussions for you and everyone else. On. For a fully mature woman, intermittent fasting will not make you feel moody, moody, irregular in the period, or otherwise because those hormones will no longer affect you, or at least, hardly. Their dietary and dietary choices are released more than the effects they have had on hormonal health over the years. Therefore, if you are trying to lose weight, better energy, a physiological shake to regain health, or whatever you have, try IF without worries and see what happens. For these types of women, intermittent fasting is set to provide hope through reduced depression, a lower chance of cancer (or recurrence), promised weight loss, and more.

Chapter 1

Intermittent Fasting For Women Over 50

There are already differences between the ways in which intermittent fasting affects men and women, so adding the difference in age makes things a little more complicated yet. Many studies related to diets and weight loss are focused on men in and around the 30 years old range. Luckily though, there are studies and resources out there for women over 50, and here I have brought them together for you to get all of the information you will need to make a safe and informed decision for your health and your body.

How Intermittent Fasting Will Affect Women Over 50 Differently

Some of the diseases or health-related issues that are more likely to affect women over the age of 50 include joint pain, arthritis, lower metabolism (which can lead to weight gain), reduced muscle mass, sleep disturbances, increased levels of belly fat, osteoporosis and other common but weight and age-related diseases such as heart disease or diabetes. By practicing intermittent fasting and losing weight; as a result, you will reduce your risk of developing several of these diseases. By inducing autophagy, you are reducing your risk of those diseases that are not as closely related to weight, such as cancer and heart attacks.

Joint Health

In women over 50, there is much more risk of developing joint issues such as knee pain, wrist, elbow, or shoulder pain. This is due to an increase in age and more risk of arthritis or low back and other joint pain due to age and overuse. In studies where women over 50 practiced intermittent fasting for a period of time, they were found to have decreased levels of joint pain, arthritic symptoms, and low back pain.

How Women Over 50 Can Benefit From Intermittent Fasting

It is quite difficult to find research that doesn't support intermittent fasting for women over 50 as an effective tool for weight loss, improved health, and better overall mental health. As long as intermittent fasting is followed in a safe manner, the results can be extremely positive!

Things for Women Over 50 to Keep in Mind

Supplementing may be very beneficial and even necessary when fasting to maintain and improve health. Some essential nutrients and minerals that your body would greatly benefit from like Omega-3's or iron may be difficult to get in adequate amounts if you are fasting. For this reason, supplementing them may benefit you in terms of keeping you feeling healthy and energetic, as well as keeping your brain functioning to its full potential. You can take specific nutrients on their own in pill-form or you can opt for a multivitamin that will include all of the most essential vitamins and minerals for overall good health. The vitamins included in a multivitamin will be those that are known to promote good overall health and those that are usually obtained through a balanced, whole food diet.

Nutrients You Need and How to Get Them

For women over the age of 50, it is important to ensure that you are getting all of the nutrients that your body needs, especially if you are trying to lose weight or are following a regime that includes fasting. To ensure that during your fasting periods, you are as healthy as possible, supplementation is something that could be considered, to ensure that you are feeding your body the nutrients it needs. It is always preferable to get the nutrients you need from whole foods rather than from supplements, but in some cases, when you cannot get everything you need from the foods in your diet alone (especially if you are eating less calories), then supplementation is always better than nothing. Below, we will look at some whole food sources as well as some supplements that you may wish to consider.

Omega 3 Fatty Acids

These are something that are essential since they cannot be made in our bodies. Omega-3 Fatty Acids are substances that are necessary to get from your diet as the body cannot make them on its own. These fatty acids are a certain type in a list of other fatty acids, but this type (Omega-3) are the most essential and the most beneficial for our brains and bodies in general. They have numerous effects on the brain including reducing inflammation (which reduces the risk of Alzheimer's) and maintaining and improving mood and cognitive function, including memory. Omega-3's have these greatly beneficial effects because of the way that they act in the brain, which is what makes them so essential to our diets. Omega-3 Fatty Acids increase the production of new nerve cells in the brain by acting specifically on the nerve stem cells within the brain, causing new and healthy nerve cells to be generated.

Omega-3 fatty acids can be found in fish like salmon, sardines, black cod, and herring. It can also be taken as a pill-form supplement for those who do not eat fish or cannot eat enough of it. It can also be taken in the form of a fish oil supplement like krill oil.

Omega-3's are by far the most important nutrient that you need to ensure you are ingesting because of the numerous benefits that come from it, both in the brain and in the rest of the body. While supplements are often a last step when it comes to trying to include something in your diet, for Omega-3's the benefits are too great to potentially miss by trying to receive all of it from your diet.

Sulphoraphane

Brussels Sprouts, Cabbage, Kale, Broccoli Sprouts have in common? All of these green vegetables have one thing in common- they all contain Sulforaphane. Sulforaphane is a plant chemical that is found naturally in these vegetables. This is an antioxidant that acts in a similar way to turmeric and thus has similar benefits. Sulforaphane like turmeric, induces autophagy in the brain which helps to reduce the risk of Alzheimer's, Parkinson's and dementia which are all neurodegenerative diseases. Neurodegenerative means that the cells in the brain called nerves are damaged and broken down, which leads to cognitive decline like Alzheimer's or physical decline as in Parkinson's. These vegetables can help to treat these diseases by slowing their progression, as they are all diseases that come about over time. There is no cure yet, but the treatment at this stage involves delaying the progression of these diseases.

Sulforaphane can be found in the aforementioned vegetables, but the strongest source is in broccoli sprouts. It can also be taken concentrated in a supplement form.

Calcium

Calcium is beneficial for the healthy circulation of blood, and for maintaining strong bones and teeth. Calcium can come from dairy products like milk, yogurt, and cheese. It can also be found in leafy greens like kale and broccoli and sardines.

Magnesium

Magnesium is beneficial for your diet, as it also helps you to maintain strong bones and teeth. Magnesium and Calcium are most effective when ingested together, as Magnesium helps in the absorption of calcium. It also helps to reduce migraines and is great for calmness and relieving anxiety. Magnesium can be found in leafy green vegetables like kale and spinach, as well as fruits like bananas and raspberries, legumes like beans and chickpeas, vegetables like peas, cabbage, green beans, asparagus and brussels sprouts, and fish like tuna and salmon.

Exogenous Ketones

When tested on animal models, even when they were ingested on a normal carbohydrate intake diet, these exogenous ketones proved to be beneficial in terms of helping the models with problems like seizures, being anti-cancer, anti-inflammation, and anti-anxiety, which are the diseases that we normally see to be assisted by ketosis (which is the state the body enters when it is using fat as a source of fuel instead of carbohydrates).

Electrolytes

When you first begin following an intermittent fasting regime, having Electrolyte depletion is quite common. This is because of water weight loss through fat and a lower carbohydrate intake, which is often common. By taking electrolyte supplements, this can help to avoid a deficiency in common electrolytes, like magnesium, potassium and sodium. This is also why you should ensure you are getting enough dietary sodium, as this is an electrolyte that you need. Along with this, though, you will need to ensure you are drinking enough water to avoid dehydration.

Iron

This one is a little tricky, but it is worth noting. Iron should be obtained in the right amounts in your diet through whole foods. If you feel like you might be deficient in iron and you are having trouble getting it in the foods you eat, you can visit your doctor for advice on this topic. Iron cannot be supplemented without being referred by a doctor first, as it is something that they would like you to first try to get from your food. If this is becoming a problem, they can give you supplements to take. This is especially a concern if you are not eating much red meat, and this may lead your doctor to want you to begin supplementing. Make an appointment with your doctor to find out more about this topic.

Vitamin D

Vitamin D is found in some foods that have been fortified with it, but in a natural sense, it can be found in only a few foods. These include cheese, fatty fish like salmon and tuna as well as egg yolks. Another source is mushrooms that have been exposed to UV rays, so the organic ones are likely of this sort.

Vitamin D can be absorbed naturally through sun exposure, so if you live in a sunny place, make sure you get out for some walks or some timer with the sun on your skin. If you live in a colder or more gloomy place, consider purchasing a lamp that mimics the sun and provides you with vitamin D in your house. On a sunny day, even if it is cold going outside and getting sun on your face will give you vitamin D.

This one is something that everyone should be conscious of, but it is especially necessary to examine if you are following a specific diet.

Bioactive Compounds

Bioactive compounds are compounds found within foods that act in the body in beneficial ways. The bioactive compounds found within berries, such as Acai Berries, Strawberries, and Blueberries are very beneficial for your health. The bioactive compounds in these specific types of berries work in the brain to induce autophagy and reduce inflammation. This leads to the protection of brain cells in this case from oxidative stress. Oxidative stress is something that can happen within the brain when there is an imbalance of oxygen, which can cause reduced cognitive functioning. These berries and their induction of autophagy helps to reduce this by keeping the balance of oxygen at a healthy level.

Chapter 2

What Are Macros?

You have probably heard the term "macronutrients" before, or at least you've heard the term "macros." In many cases, you will hear people on the ketogenic diet talking about them because tracking them is a huge part of that regimen. Tracking your macros should be a huge part of just about any regimen, regardless of it being ketogenic or not.

Macronutrients are, quite simply, the nutritional compounds or elements that you're putting into your body when you eat. The most common ones to watch are protein, carbohydrates, and fats. The reason for looking at these is to make sure that you're keeping things in an adequate balance in your diet. If you're eating mostly fat without eating enough protein or enough carbohydrates, your body will react differently. If you know you need to be eating a certain amount of protein each day, then you will keep a keener eye out for the things that have more of it like chicken breasts, or other lean meats, as they will add protein without adding considerable fat.

In most cases, there aren't rigid numbers you need to stick for each of these while doing intermittent fasting. It is important, however, that you're not taking on foods that are mostly carbs or fat while you're dieting, right? If you want to make sure that your body is going to get the most out of the things you're eating without feeling sluggish or putting on excess weight, you're not going to be eating things that are primarily carbohydrates either.

Carbohydrates

Your body will primarily use carbs as its means of fuel and most typical diets will dictate that you make up your diet with about 45%-65% carbs. Your body will use carbohydrates as the fuel for just about every internal process it has. Your body can very easily break down carbohydrates, making it a convenient fuel source when taken on in the right amounts. There are some doctor-recommended programs for those who need to reduce their weight that require that this percentage be drastically reduced, but that's not typical.

Carbohydrates, when they break down, are converted into glucose, which is the real raw fuel your body can use to keep moving. Glucose is absorbed into the cells of your body, fueling each one's processes. When your body ends up with an excess of glucose, it gets converted once more into something else called glycogen which is converted into the fat stores your body keeps for future use. This is sort of an evolutionary holdover that allows you to get through periods of starvation, as food was far scarcer than it is today. However, most of us are in no position to starve and those fat stores stick around doing no good for anyone until we work them off.

One of the things to bear in mind when you're evaluating whether or not to cut carbohydrates is that there is no one type of carbohydrate and that deciding "carbs are bad," is not as black and white or correct as it might seem. There are simple carbohydrates and there are complex carbohydrates.

The labels "simple" and "complex" refer to the length of the molecule itself, which is obviously not something you'll be able to tell just by looking at the food. You will, however, be able to know it by whether or not the food is processed. Simple carbohydrates that take your body almost no time to burn through and your body will typically be left with more glycogen at the end of that process. Complex carbohydrates take a longer time to break down in the body and give your body more fuel in the time it takes to break them down.

Simple carbohydrates are mostly sugars, so you'll find those in candies, sodas, juices, and things like that. Complex carbohydrates are in things like bananas, legumes, and whole grains.

There is no black and white answer about whether simple or complex carbs are better or worse for you, but you will generally find that complex carbs are much better for *lasting power*. You will, however, find that if you avoid processed foods, you will feel better and get the most out of the carbs that you do eat!

Protein

Proteins are used to build muscle and repair the body to keep it going from day to day. That's why you need more protein if you decide to start working out and exercising more. Your body needs to recuperate and repair and protein is the ideal helper for that process. It's recommended that about 20%-35% of your daily intake is made up of proteins.

The protein that you take on allows your body to restore cells, to grow, to grow your hair and nails, to repair and refresh your skin, and all that very essential stuff! This doesn't mean that eating 100% protein will help your body regenerate like a comic book character, but it does mean that it's quite important to ensure that you're getting enough protein!

You get essential amino acids from the foods that you eat, and those will often come from the animal proteins that you eat. There are 20 amino acids and nine of those aren't produced in our bodies. They're classified as essential because we need to get them from the foods that we eat, namely the animal proteins. If you're a vegetarian, you can get them from sources of plant-based protein.

Fat

Over the decades, you've likely watched the stigma and public opinion surrounding fats evolve. For a while, every diet food was fat-free, then there was the Atkins craze and food couldn't have enough fat in it to satisfy shoppers and dieters, and it's been an ever-evolving cycle ever since. Without getting too confusing about the truth of fats, here is the long and short of it. Fats should take up about 10%-35% of your daily intake. Of those fats, you want to make sure that as many as possible are "good fats."

This means you want fats from lean protein sources, fats that contain Omega-3 fatty acids, Omega-6 fatty acids, and which don't come from overly processed foods. These come from things like fish, walnuts, eggs, and vegetable oils. When foods naturally have fat in them without any help from processes like homogenization or emulsification, you will generally find the fats to be good. The fats in dairy are helpful to the body in moderation, and if you aren't lactose intolerant.

You can also look for these things:

Saturated Fats – These come from meat, dairy, and other animal byproducts.

Unsaturated Fats – These are the plant-based fats that come from veggies, nuts, and the like.

Trans Fats – These types of fats are generally only produced in the commercial production and processing of foods like fast foods, snack foods, and butter substitutes that aren't plant-based.

Trans fats should be avoided for the most part, if not entirely, as those are fats your body can't particularly use and which don't contribute to healthy heart function.

What Should My Macros be During Intermittent Fasting?

There is no set amount of each macro that you should be taking on each day when you're doing intermittent fasting. You will find that you generally want to keep to the percentages outlined above for your macros. That means that you should be eating enough to fill you up without going overboard. In many cases, you will lose weight on intermittent fasting because you won't eat as much as you otherwise would.

Those macros once again are:

Carbs: 45% to 65%

Protein: 20% to 35%

Fats: 10% to 35%

If you are able to make sure your macros are just about in this range, then you will often find that you are feeling your best and that you are doing quite well. If you need the help of a calorie-tracking app, you might find that you're more able to stay on top of your intake and that you're able to feel fuller for longer without overdoing it.

It's not completely necessary to watch your calories in order to do intermittent fasting and to feel the benefits that it has to offer, but it can help you to keep on track and to keep yourself from doing things you wish you hadn't. You might even find that some of your favorite foods are even better for you than you had initially anticipated!

Unfortunately, many of us are not familiar with serving sizes and how much of things we're supposed to be eating in a sitting. Many of us have taken out cues from the restaurants around us and, the horrible truth is that the average restaurant will serve you 2-3 times as much as you're supposed to be eating in one sitting!

If you have found yourself wondering why you're not losing weight when you think you've been eating everything in moderation, it could be worth it to track your calorie and food intake on one of those apps to see what you're really taking in.

Chapter 3

Types of Intermittent Fasting

The 16/8 Method

This is one of the most common methods that you can use in intermittent fasting. During this method you have to fast for about 14 to 16 hours each day, and eat the rest of the hours. During this feeding time, you can still take in two to three meals with no problem. This is more likely to fit in with the lunch schedule that you're used to, but it still affects you so you don't eat all day.

This approach is simpler than you'd expect. After dinner it's as easy as not eating meals and then skipping breakfast or at least having a late snack. Okay, you're just fasting for 16 hours because you're finishing your last meal at 8 o'clock in the night, and then eating nothing until midday the next day. Just be careful of the late-night therapies. Eating them in the morning will require you to skip coffee.

Many people have issues with this because in the morning they feel hungry for food and they know they need to sleep. Only shift the meal to a bit later in the day. If you choose, for example, to eat breakfast at 10 a.m. You would still be within the 16-hour period instead of eight, and then stop eating at 6 a.m.

As a woman, this form of intermittent fasting is advisable. With these shorter fasts, women typically do well and it is best to go fasting for 14 to 15 hours as this is more helpful to you.

During the quick, you are allowed to drink beer, tea, coffee and other non-caloric liquids to help lessen hunger pains. In fact, you should try to stick to healthier foods during your feeding time. Eating a lot of unsanitary food during this time isn't a good idea. Many people like to have a low-carb diet when they are on a fast intermittent because it deals with fatigue and gives better outcomes.

The rationale behind the approach of 16/8 focuses on your hormonal rhythms and biological clock. According to Satchidananda Panda, a professor at the Salk Institute for Biological Studies and an expert in the field of biology and circadian rhythms, the body has not only one biological clock but several which make up the full circadian rhythm. There's one biological clock in your liver, one in your kidneys and one in your stomach, and according to Panda, each of these clocks were switched on and turned off at various times.

Shortly after you feed the digestive system kicks in gear. When food moves through your digestive tract, every organ involved in the digestive process turns on, eats the food, and then turns off. When all digestive organs are shut off, it will allow the digestive system time to rest. During this time, the digestive system does its own "cleanup"— similar to a concept of a self-cleaning oven. Any remaining food residues are cleaned out, and the body is ready to start over again.

And if you constantly put food in your mouth, it will never shut down your digestive system, so it will never have enough time to perform its self-cleaning, which will have a negative impact on both your metabolism and overall health. Through his study, Panda found that giving the body an eight to twelve-hour, no-food window is best for your health. He claims it will help you lose weight (or maintain a healthy weight) and help stave off diabetes, high cholesterol and obesity by introducing a daily fasting period.

The Importance of Your Circadian Rhythm

For fully understand Panda's work, it is helpful to know what your circadian rhythm is, and how it affects the body. Also referred to as a body clock or biological clock, the circadian rhythm is a twenty-four-hour cycle that regulates many of the body's physiological processes, including sleep and digestion. The body gets signals from your circadian rhythm about when to go to sleep, when to wake up and when to feed.

Your circadian rhythm is regulated centrally by a brain area called the hypothalamus but is primarily influenced by natural, environmental signals such as temperature and light. For example, when it's dark outside, your eyes send a signal to your hypothalamus that it's time for you to sleep; your hypothalamus sends a message to the pineal gland (in another area of your brain) that activates melatonin (a hormone that helps you sleep), and you get sleepy. When it is light-out the opposite happens. Your eyes send your hypothalamus a signal, sending a signal to your pineal gland to reduce the production of melatonin. A dip in melatonin will make you stand up and get ready for the day.

The 5:2 diet

The 5:2 diet is another viable option. This fast advises you to eat normally for five days during the week and to limit yourself for each of the other two days to no more than 600 calories. This is sometimes called the Easy Diet, too.

It's recommended that on these fasting days, people will eat around 500 calories. You'll normally eat every day of the week, for example, and on Monday and Thursdays you'll have only two small meals with at least 500 calories. You can choose any day of the week as your fasting days, as long as you don't have them back to back. Choose your two busy days of the week, and make them fasting days.

There aren't many reports out there about the 5:2 diet, but it will provide most of the benefits you're finding as it's intermittent fast. You can do it without the need to think all day about making meals.

Eat-Stop-Eat diet

The Eat-Stop-Eat diet helps you skip 24-hour meals once or twice a week. This method was first popularized by Brad Pilon and has been a popular way to do the sporadic quickly for some time. You can do this quickly while still having one meal a day. Some citizens will have dinner every day, and then eat nothing until the supper of the next day. It lets you never go a whole day without eating but still collapsing in the 24-hour abstinence process.

You do want to change that though. You can choose one of those options when going from breakfast to breakfast or lunch to lunch is best for you. During your fast, you are allowed to have coffee, water, and other non-caloric drinks to keep you hydrated but you are not permitted to have any food at all.

Note that you're just fasting for one or two days a week. If it's time to eat properly, you need to consume the same amount of food you would have if you weren't on a fast. This will help you lose weight without hurting your body.

The only problem with getting on with this kind of erratic fast is that working for 24 hours is hard for most people. Nonetheless, you can ease that in it. You can find that beginning with a shorter speed, like the 16-hour fast, can produce some good results, and then continue to run for longer periods of time. Without food it can be hard to go through a whole day and most people tend to go with one of the other fasting options to see the same effects.

Alternate day fasting

With this choice, -alternate day you'll go on a fast. You can take with you a few things, and it depends on what applies to your needs. Some of those fasts that would allow you to have around 500 calories on your fasting days. You will find that most sporadic laboratory studies used some version of the simple alternate day to help determine all health benefits. Every other day it can be daunting to most people to fast.

It's certainly something you'll need to build up to every other day. It can be a struggle to push yourself to eat on alternate days. You'll probably feel very hungry many days a week on this fasting schedule, and it's hard to stick to that over the long run.

Warrior Diet

The warrior's way of fasting is remaining hungry for the entire day and then eating food at night. This can work well for people who are workaholics and do not have time to eat. This can also be very useful for people who are traveling far. Eating in a journey can be difficult and unwanted for a few people. If you train your body for the warrior diet, then you can easily skip eating during a long journey.

You can however have small portions of fruits and vegetables that are healthy during the day. Do not eat anything heavy though. For the warrior method of fasting, you get a 4 hours window to eat anything during the night.

Since it is called the warrior diet, you also should eat like how our warriors of ancient times used to eat, "unprocessed food". You should only eat foods that are not processed; basically "whole food" is the way to go with this method. Warrior fasting method is quite similar to the food choices we have in the "paleo diet".

Spontaneous Meal Skipping

You should do this if you want to prep your body for intermittent fasting, or if you don't want to spend a lot of time worrying about when you can drink. With this easy, you don't need to worry about following one of the more organized, intermittent fasting programs. You'll probably miss any meals occasionally. If you are not thirsty, or if you are too exhausted for a meal, you can do this. It is a big myth that you have to eat food every few hours to stop hunger.

The liver is well adapted without food, to last long periods. Waiting on a few meals isn't harmful to your health, particularly if you're not hungry or too busy.

If you end up eating a meal, or two, you are actually fasting. If you are too busy to get a snack out of the door just make sure you eat a good lunch and dinner. When you run out of errands and can't find a place to eat, then it's great to miss out on a snack. It will do no good and will really save you money.

You probably won't see results as good as some of the other options, but it's better than nothing and it's much easier to work with. Perhaps try skipping one or two meals during the week, or missing any meals when it's going for you.

As you can see, there are several different options you can deal with when you're ready to go on the sporadic quick. Some of these will be simpler than others and some will fit your timetable better. You'll need to choose which pace to work in your everyday life is best.

Extended Fasting

Although extended fasting belongs to one class of its own, it is important to understand the difference between it and the other types of intermittent fasting. Extended fasting is any form of fast that lasts longer than 24 hours. Long fasting can often last for a week and many of these long fasts simply require drinking liquids.

These types of fasts are more normal throughout the medical and surgical settings and are usually done when the body needs to experience substantial recovery or when the ability to feed is impaired. Without the guidance and monitoring of a medical professional, you should not pursue a continuous pace.

Chapter 4

Autophagy

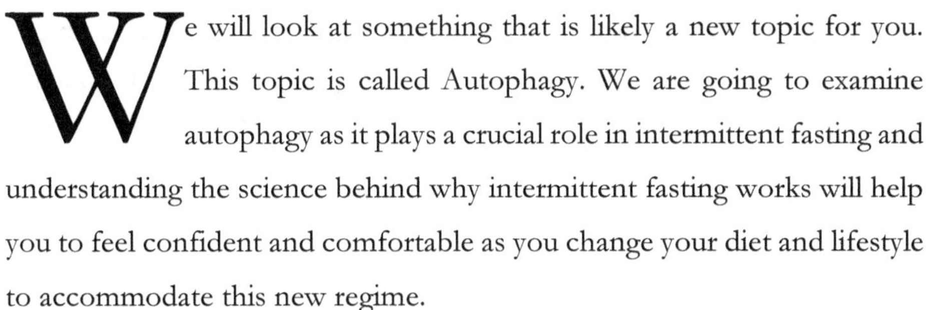

We will look at something that is likely a new topic for you. This topic is called Autophagy. We are going to examine autophagy as it plays a crucial role in intermittent fasting and understanding the science behind why intermittent fasting works will help you to feel confident and comfortable as you change your diet and lifestyle to accommodate this new regime.

What is Autophagy

Autophagy itself is a process that happens within the body, and that has been going on since the beginning of humans. It is only recently that people began harnessing this process to achieve desired positive results. We will look at this topic in-depth throughout this book but here we will begin by looking at what exactly Autophagy is.

Autophagy, as a word, can be broken up into two individual parts. Each of these parts on its own is a separate Greek word. The word auto, which means self and the word phagy which means the practice of eating. Putting these together gives you the practice of self-eating, which is essentially what autophagy is. Now this may sound like some type of new-age cannibalism, but it is a very natural process that our cells practice all the time without us being any the wiser. Autophagy is the body's way of cleaning itself out.

The process of autophagy involves small "hunter" particles that go around your body, looking for cells or cell components that are old and damaged. The hunter particles then take these cell components apart, getting rid of the damaged parts and saving the useful parts to make new cells later. These hunter cells can also use the leftover useful parts to create energy for the body.

Autophagy has been found to happen in all organisms that are multi-cellular, like animals and plants, in addition to humans. While the study of these larger organisms and how autophagy works in their cells is lesser-known, more studies are being done on humans and how changes in diet can affect their body's autophagy.

The other function that autophagy serves is that it helps cells to carry out their death when it is time for them to die. There are times when cells are programmed to die, because of a number of different factors. Sometimes these cells need assistance in their death, and autophagy can help them with this or can help to clean up after their death. The human body is all about life and death and these processes are continually going on without our knowledge to keep us healthy and in good form.

As I mentioned, the process of autophagy has been going on inside of us for many, many years, since the beginning of humans. This process has been kept around inside of our bodies because of the multitude of benefits it can provide us with. It is also essential for the health of our bodies, as being able to get rid of waste and damaged parts that are no longer useful to us is essential to our health. If we were unable to get rid of damaged or broken cells, these damaged particles would build up and eventually make us sick. Our bodies are extremely efficient in everything that they do, and waste disposal is no different.

It is in more recent years that the study of autophagy has been focused more heavily on in terms of diet and disease research. These studies are still in their early stages as it has been only a few years shy of sixty years since autophagy was discovered. This process was discovered in a lab by testing what happened when small organisms went without food for some time. These organisms were observed very closely under a microscope, and it was found that their cells had this process of waste disposal and energy creation that was later named autophagy.

More about autophagy and its relation to energy production is being studied in recent years, as this topic is of interest to humans. Autophagy can use old cell parts and recycle them to create new energy that the organism (like the human or animal) can then use to do its regular functions like walking and breathing. Now, people are studying what happens when humans rely on this form of energy production instead of the energy they would get from ingesting food throughout the day. This is where autophagy and intermittent fasting come together. We will look at how they work together throughout the rest of this book as we delve deeply into intermittent fasting and autophagy and how they work together to allow for things like weight loss or disease prevention.

What is the Function of Autophagy?

Autophagy has many functions in the body. "What is autophagy," you learned that it is a process that helps to discard old and damaged cells and use their parts for energy. We will look at some of the other functions of autophagy and the body systems involved.

Autophagy is said to be the housekeeping function of the body. If you think of your body as your home, autophagy is the housekeeper that you hire to take care of all of the waste and the recycling functions of your cells.

One of the housekeeping duties includes removing cell parts that were built wrongly or at the wrong time. Sometimes cells make mistakes, and these mistakes can cause proteins or other cell parts to be formed in error. When this happens, we need something within the cell to get rid of these so that they do not take up space or get in the way of other processes within the cell. Further, sometimes useful parts of the cell will become damaged somehow and then will need to be removed in order to make way for a new part to take its place. These cell parts can include those that create DNA or those that create the proteins needed to make the DNA.

Another duty of autophagy is to protect the body from disease and pathogens. Pathogens are bacteria or viruses that can infect our cells and our bodies if they are not properly defended against. Autophagy works to kill the cells within our body that are infected by these pathogens in order to get rid of them before they can spread. In this way, autophagy plays a part in our immune system as it acts as a supplement to our immune cells whose sole function is to protect us from invasions by disease and infection.

Autophagy also functions to help the cells of the body to regulate themselves when there are stressors placed upon them. These stressors can be things like a lack of food for the cell or physical stresses placed on the cell. This regulation helps to maintain a standard cell environment despite factors that can change, like the availability of food. Autophagy is able to do things like break down cell parts for food to provide the cell with nutrients.

Similar to its role in regulation of the cells, autophagy also helps with the development of a growing fetus inside of a woman's uterus. Autophagy occurs here to ensure that the embryo has enough nutrients and energy at all times for healthy development. In addition to this, it helps with growth in adults as well as there is a balance of building new parts and breaking down old ones involved in the growth of any organism.

Autophagy is more important than we may even realize, as it plays a large role in the survival of the living organisms it acts within. It does this by being especially sensitive to the levels of nutrients and energy within a cell. When the nutrient levels lower, autophagy breaks down cell parts which create nutrients and energy for the cell. If it weren't for this process, the cells would not be able to maintain their ideal functioning environment and they may begin to make more mistakes and even lower their functioning abilities altogether. So much goes on inside of a cell that they need to be able to work effectively at all times. Autophagy makes this possible which is what makes it such an essential function.

How Does Autophagy Work in the Body

Autophagy functions in the following way. When a decrease in nutrients is noticed within a cell, this decrease in nutrients acts as a signal for the cell to create small pockets within a membrane (a thin barrier layer) that are called autophagosomes. These small pockets (autophagosomes) move through the cell and find debris and damaged particles floating around within the cell. The small pockets then consume this debris by absorbing it into its inner space. The debris is then enclosed in the membrane (the thin barrier layer) and is moved to a place in the cell called the Lysosome. A lysosome is a part of a cell that acts as a center for degradation, breakdown, or disassembly. This part of the cell gets debris and damaged cell parts delivered to it by the autophagosomes. Once these damaged cell parts are delivered, the lysosomes then break them down. By breaking them down, these parts can be recycled and used for energy.

Two Types of Autophagy

There are two different forms of autophagy- Macroautophagy and Microautophagy. These two different types act in slightly different ways.

Macroautophagy

For the most part, when you hear or see the word autophagy, it is in reference to *Macroautophagy*. This is the form that is most often discussed in relation to things like diet and health.

Microautophagy

Microautophagy differs from Macroautophagy slightly in the way that it works. While both still accomplish the same end goal, the way that they get there is what sets them apart from each other. In the type of autophagy, small pockets surrounded by membranes called autophagosomes are created, and they take up debris in the cell and move it to the lysosomes to be broken down and used for energy. When it comes to Microautophagy, the difference is that the debris floating around within the cell moves to the lysosome on its own without being carried there inside of an autophagosome. Once it reaches the lysosome, it is engulfed by the membrane of the lysosome and then is taken inside to be broken down.

Sometimes the way that this debris reaches the lysosome in Microautophagy is not totally on its own, as there is a protein complex that escorts or chaperones it to the lysosome. If there is a signal of low nutrient levels within the cell and Microautophagy is needed in addition to Macroautophagy, then the chaperone proteins may search out debris within the cell and escort it to the lysosome to be taken inside. The chaperone protein will then leave to find more debris to escort back to the lysosome.

Macroautophagy versus Microautophagy

Now that you know that there are two different types of autophagy and the difference between them, you may be wondering which one occurs when and which of these two we are more concerned with when it comes to disease and health.

Both of these processes are occurring regularly within our cells, and the frequency with which each of them occurs must create a balance. This balance must be created for one very important reason. When the small pockets called autophagosomes are created and they move to the lysosome, they attach their membrane to the membrane of the lysosome in order to drop off the debris that they contain. Then, once the debris is dropped off, this new membrane that has attached itself is left there, thus becoming a part of the membrane of the lysosome. This increases the size of the lysosome membrane by a bit of length each time. When Microautophagy occurs, the debris meets the outside of the lysosome and is taken into the lysosome by being engulfed by the membrane of the lysosome which creates a small pocket inside of the lysosome that contains the debris. This new small pocket has been created by the lysosome membrane, meaning that the lysosome membrane has become shorter in length by a small amount. Because of the way these two types of autophagy act, they must happen at about the same frequency as each other so that the size of the lysosome membrane can remain consistent. If this was not the case, we would either be left with a much larger lysosome due to increased lysosome membrane size after Macroautophagy, or a much smaller lysosome in the case of Microautophagy. These two processes not only ensure that the lysosome size remains consistent, but they ensure that the debris within the cell is broken down and recycled as efficiently as possible.

Chapter 5

Growing Old Gracefully and Gradually

—•◦•—

Growing old gracefully I would imagine is the ambition of most women. In some cultures, the aged members of the community are respected, revered, and held in high esteem. Younger members of the community often seek their knowledge and advice. The hierarchy of age in many communities carries authority and responsibility and their position is aspired to by younger members of the clan. The elders are treated with care, empathy, and deference until they die.

In Western culture, however, youth is often glorified, while age is considered contemptible and is all too often ignored. The sad outcome of this behavior towards the aged members of our society is that many of these bright, alert, and knowledgeable elderly people end up maligned and alone, struggling to come to terms with the fact that they no longer have value or a purpose in life.

Many people are afraid of dying and facing the unknown after death. The majority of people who are currently fit, healthy, and strong would like to continue their lives for as long as possible, so they make adequate and sensible plans to achieve their goals. With the immense advances in scientific research and medical technology, modern humans have a myriad of potential life-lengthening support systems at their fingertips. The secret is, of course, to make timeous adjustments to your current lifestyle if you want to enjoy a youthful, energetic old age.

Age Is Determined in a Number of Ways

So how is age actually determined? You may know of people who, although well into their senior years are still leading active, healthy lives, while others who are a great deal younger, already appear old and frail. What makes some of us appear older or younger than we really are?

Age is measured in three specific ways and together these results determine just how old you actually are.

Chronological age:

Your chronological age is linked to the number of years you have been alive. Although it may have no relevance to the individual's overall health, it may be a useful tool that can be used for long-term financial planning and making decisions about your future. However, as you age, the chances of health problems begin to increase. Many of these changes in your health may creep up unexpectedly. It is this slow and insidious decline in your health that leads to the onset of old age. So, the healthier and fitter you are throughout your life, the more likely you will be able to enjoy your senior years.

Biological age:

Your biological age refers to the normal, expected age-related changes to your body and mind at any given age. Some people experience an earlier onset of old age than others. This event is primarily due to individual lifestyles, eating habits, personal outlook on life, physical fitness levels, and of course the unexpected onset of disease. Some people exhibit the symptoms of agedness before the biologically considered old age of 65, while other people may still be active and lead healthy lives for at least another 10 to 12 years.

Psychological age:

Your psychological age is based on how you behave and feel. This has nothing to do with your age in years but has more to do with your mental and emotional outlook on life. Your psychological age contributes to your willingness to participate in events in your life, such as continuing to work, taking an active interest in supporting a specific charity by doing voluntary work, taking up a new and interesting hobby or joining a group of like-minded people for regular, thought-provoking and inspiring meetings. It is your psychological age that takes control of your outlook on life and promotes a positive or negative attitude toward aging (Besdine, 2019).

Normal Aging as Opposed to Dementia

As with all living organisms, humans age both internally and externally. The external signs of growing older are visible in wrinkles and graying hair, perhaps a slower gait and some difficulty with vision, hearing, and possibly memory loss. There may also be a decline in your ability to concentrate and stay focused on a topic for a specific amount of time.

The rate at which people age internally has not yet been scientifically proven, but the general trend appears to include a slowing down of bodily functions and sometimes a slow impairment of your senses and skills.

Dementia sufferers are generally classed as elderly and although their chronological age may be younger than other people, their mind and brain have aged significantly. Scientific studies have shown a marked difference in the brain tissue of normally aging people with that of people suffering from Alzheimer's disease (Besdine, 2019).

Why is it then that the aging process appears to affect specific people in different ways? The general consensus is that the aging process is directly linked to our individual lifestyles and the potential conclusion is that the healthier and more active we are, the more likely we will be to grow old happily and gracefully.

Healthy Aging

Healthy aging refers to your ability to postpone or reduce the effects of the aging process in some sensible, healthy ways. These include:

- •following a healthy, nutritious diet,

- •doing regular, sensible exercise, and

- •staying mentally active and alerts.

Women approaching their 50s who wish to make the best of their senior years will benefit from seriously considering changing their lifestyle and habits to include the above suggestions.

Richard W. Besdine at the Warren Alpert Medical School of Brown University reports there is some evidence of a definite increase in healthy aging in the USA. This is due to the following:

- •Despite the increase in persons over the age of 65 and 85 still being alive and active, there are fewer of these individuals living in nursing homes or requiring supportive care. Many of these people remain active and independent for longer.

- •There has been a noticeable decrease in people between the ages of 75 and 84 with reported impairments, such as hearing or vision loss.
- •A marked drop in the number of individuals over the age of 65 who are suffering from debilitating disorders such as dementia, and Alzheimer's, has been noted.

Increased Life Expectancy

The life expectancy of the average citizen in the U.S. has increased extensively during the past century. Female children born during the 1900s were expected to live no longer than about 46 years, while those who were born in the 2000s have an increased life expectancy of at least 81+ years.

The reasons for these distinct changes in people's life expectancy is partly due to the dramatic advancement in medical technology and education as well as their access to vast amounts of valuable information about nutrition, physical fitness, and an overall healthier lifestyle (Besdine, 2019).

Ten Important Suggestions for Growing Old Gracefully

Pay regular visits to your doctor

Girls, now that you are in your 50s, you may often experience nagging health matters, including unusual aches and pains, dizziness, nausea, abnormal bodily functions, growths, bruising and breathlessness, to name but a few. Be proactive rather than neglectful and ensure your annual physical is up to date. The sooner these symptoms are checked out and where needed, medicated, the sooner you will be back on top and able to enjoy your life. After all, you are at the age when you want to live your life to the fullest, so don't let the check-ups slide!

You are what you eat!

As you age, your metabolism begins to change around the onset of middle-age, and it behooves you to consider altering your food and drink intake accordingly. Enjoying good food and drinks is an important aspect of many fortunate people's lives and during your youth, you may not have taken much notice of the type of food you ingested. You burn fewer calories as you age because you may not be as active as you were when you were younger. Although a well-balanced diet is of paramount importance to your longevity, your meal portion size should begin to diminish as you grow older. It is, however, important to remember the rule, 'everything in moderation'.

The importance of rest and the value of meditation

During your youth, you probably spent most of your time working to achieve all that you now enjoy. Around the age of retirement, some people may begin to panic and wonder how they will cope with all the free time they will have when they stop working.

Added to this are the very real worries about your financial status when you retire. Some people are fortunate enough to have made adequate plans for their old age, while others are not so lucky. Stress in any form has a negative impact on not only your health but your sleep patterns.

Adequate rest cannot be overemphasized. It forms an essential part of your healthy lifestyle and goes a long way to promote the control of the secretion of hormones beneficial to the development and maintenance of your immune system, appetite, energy levels, mental acuity, and a general sense of well-being.

Another way in which you can enjoy rest and relaxation is through mindful meditation. Daily meditation is not only good for the soul but also has a powerful, decisive effect on your ability to tune into the positive aspects of your life and to express your gratitude for all your blessings. It also plays a positive role in retaining your good memory and aiding digestion.

Have the confidence to try new things

Being fabulous and 50 and possibly preparing to retire does not mean your life no longer has value and purpose. Women over 50 can benefit hugely from learning new skills and perhaps starting an interesting new hobby. It is vitally important to be willing to try new things and to bring some enjoyment and fun into your life. The company of others and your participation in group activities will ensure you do not stagnate and lose interest in life. You may need reminding that you are a special and wonderful individual, so consider planning something special to look forward to each day.

Take care of your appearance

All women should take a keen interest in their appearance and treat themselves with respect. However, as you mature and begin to age it is important to view yourself less critically and to learn to be content with who you have become. Wrinkles and lines on your face and body are part of the aging process. Rather than deny these changes in your physical self, embrace them as signs of your life's experiences and wisdom. Self-acceptance brings a great deal of inner peace and tranquility to the soul and mind. In turn, these qualities can instill you with a more positive self-image and enable you to face each day with growing enthusiasm and grace.

Connect with people

Growing old can sometimes be a lonely experience. Many elderly people live alone and may seldom enjoy contact with other people. Women, in particular, are social beings who benefit from the company of others. So do not hesitate to reach out to people of a similar age to make new friends. It is important to maintain and grow your social and communication skills by sharing new ideas and listening attentively to others in your own companionable group. By positively interacting with people, you increase your chances of maintaining a more youthful and happier outlook on life.

Recalling your youth

Although it is neither a healthy nor worthwhile diversion to dwell on your past, it is important to recall and rejoice in all the happy and successful times you have had the good fortune to experience. Reminiscing is a wonderful way of reliving past events and recalling happy memories that can positively impact your own youthful feelings and emotions. However, try to avoid becoming bogged down by negative memories as these can tarnish your present state by filling you with sadness and regret.

Plan an exciting trip

Sitting around at home alone is definitely not good for anyone's health and mental strength and will in no way assist you in fulfilling your 'bucket list'. It may take a great deal of courage for you to get out as often as you are able. Falling into a 'rut' and becoming home-bound is certainly not a good plan. Unless you are totally incapacitated, try inviting a friend to join you and visit new places and meet new people. Even if you are unable to travel far, take short trips to places that interest you and learn something about each place you visit. By adding some excitement to your life, you are more likely to keep yourself young at heart and feel more positive about your life.

Take on the responsibility of caring for a pet

Owning a pet encourages most people to step out of their comfort zone once in a while. Animals accept their humans for who they are. They don't care about their owner's looks, height, weight or wealth. Their unconditional love and loyalty encompass their human caregivers creating an often unbreakable bond between a pet and its owner. Sadly, there are some retirement homes that do not allow pets. However, if you are able to, consider getting yourself a pet. Although the choice of animal is yours, you may find yourself drawn to the 'frosty' members at the pet care shelter. Older animals seldom have the chance of being adopted by young families, and so these wonderful animals often make perfect pets for retired people.

If you cannot keep a pet of your own, consider becoming a volunteer at a local pet shelter. You will not only be helping the organization with some of its daily chores, but you will also have the valuable opportunity to bond with some of the animals at the shelter.

Your opinion is very important

Being a member of the fabulous 50s age group affords you the opportunity to take your courage in both hands and stand up for what you believe in. As you age, you learn there are many times when you can speak up. Take advantage of these opportunities to voice your opinion, offer advice or make suggestions. Many people may not consider your words of any value, but there will be those who seek and value your input and comment (Koopman, 2015).

And remember, age is just a number. You are only as old as you believe yourself to be. So go out into the world with a positive outlook and be the guiding light for someone who may need a mentor or a friend.

Chapter 6

Advantages and Disadvantages of Intermittent Fasting

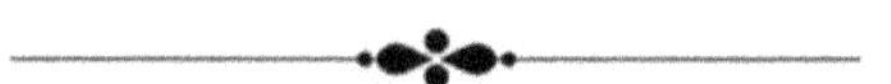

There are pros and cons to every lifestyle. For instance, when you are eating a healthy and nutritious diet, you may lose weight and gain health but be unable to eat all your favorite foods in the amount you would like. On the other hand, when you eat junk food all the time you may enjoy yourself, but you will lose health and gain weight. In the same way, there are naturally both pros and cons to intermittent fasting, and by understanding what they are, you can better manage your lifestyle. Like all things, you will find that these pros and cons are most evened out when intermittent fasting is done in moderation. If a person only rarely practices fasting, then they will, in turn, only experience a few of the benefits. On the other hand, if they practice intermittent fasting overly enthusiastically and for longer periods than healthy, then they will experience more of the drawbacks.

Thankfully, with a balanced intermittent fasting schedule, you can find yourself experiencing many of the benefits and few, if any, of the drawbacks.

While some pros and cons of intermittent fasting are universal, others can be affected by gender and age. We will be exploring what pros and cons you individually may experience as a woman in or over her fifties.

Advantages of Intermittent Fasting

Boost Weight Loss

Most people discover intermittent fasting either because they want to lose weight or gain health benefits. But, sometimes losing weight can accomplish both of those simultaneously, as a high body fat percentage can increase high blood pressure, cholesterol, and early mortality. Whether you are hoping to gain these health benefits by losing weight or wish to lose weight to feel more comfortable in your skin, you will love the way that intermittent fasting can boost your weight loss.

Balance Important Hormones

Thankfully, studies have found intermittent fasting can help balance a person's cortisol and melioration levels. It does this in a variety of ways. For instance, it can help to reduce cortisol by balancing and regulating blood sugar levels. By balancing cortisol, it sets off a chain reaction that improves the balance of other hormones, including melatonin. One simple change can benefit many hormones and systems within your body.

Improve Heart Health

As we age, we all must take even more care of our heart health. After all, heart disease is the number one killer of both men and women. While most often doctors educate men on the symptoms and warning signs of heart attacks, women are often forgotten, leading to increased risk of death. This means women must be extra vigilant, taking care of their heart health and educating themselves on the warning signs of heart attacks.

One crucial way to increase heart health is to watch your cholesterol. There is not a single type of cholesterol, but several. The two main types include LDL, which is known as the "bad" cholesterol, and HDL, known as the "good" cholesterol. While LDL cholesterol will increase your risk of heart attack and heart disease, HDL cholesterol will protect your heart health and remove LDL cholesterol from your body.

Increase Mental Energy and Efficiency

We all need mental energy to get through the day. When our mind is sluggish, we are unable to think, accomplish anything, and sometimes we may be unable even to stay awake. We have all had troubles at times focusing on work, completing a math problem, remembering what we have read, and so on. This is all due to a lack of mental energy and efficiency. You may think that intermittent fasting would further reduce your mental state, as hunger makes focusing difficult, but the opposite is exact.

Reduce the Potential Risk of Developing Cancer

Of course, nobody can promise that any lifestyle choice will prevent you from developing cancer in the future. However, studies have found that intermittent fasting can potentially reduce your risk. Further studies are ongoing, but current research through animal studies have proven promising. For instance, it was found that rats with tumors survive longer when placed on fasting schedules than the control group.

Increase Longevity

Early studies on animals have found that by including intermittent fasting, an animal can experience an increased lifespan. These studies found that even if animals had a higher body fat percentage than the control group, by including intermittent fasting, they were able to increase their lifespan and longevity.

This makes sense, as intermittent fasting has many health benefits, and when all of these benefits are compounded together, it naturally results in a longer lifespan.

Lifestyle Ease

We all want improving health and weight, but it is important also to have an easier lifestyle. When it is difficult to gain health and weight, many of us end up failing, as life is already busy and difficult enough without adding added worry and tasks. If a person cook more, eat more frequently, and always worry about a diet, they are unlike to stick to it, as it is merely is unmaintainable.

It supports the secretion of the growth hormone.

It's present in kids more than in grown-ups, but it still helps a lot. The growth hormone decreases fat and improves the development of bone and muscles. It does this by turning glycogen to glucose into the bloodstream. This enables fat burn without the reduction of muscles. When you sleep and exercise enough, the growth hormone is also boosted.

It enables you to avoid heart illnesses.

Both blood glucose control and fat loss are done by IF improve heart health. The likelihood of getting coronary artery heart illness can also be reduced.

Intermittent fasting is very versatile and can fit in any schedule.

It is not as challenging as certain diets that unnecessarily trigger a huge disturbance in your life. There is no particular time to perform the IF. They can be blended as you think it is appropriate for your timetable. You are not boxed into any regiment that you cannot retain easily. Intermittent rapidity adapts to life's unpredictability. This can also be practiced everywhere in the globe as there is no special gear you need so as to do it; it only restricts your feeding and is therefore much easier and more practical than many diets. It's completely all right, even if you have to halt fasting for a while. In a matter of minutes, you can begin fasting again.

It accepts all food

Organic foods have more nutrients than processed foods. These organic products are unfortunately quite costly, so purchasing them will diminish your pockets every day. In fact, they can be almost 10 times more expensive than processed products. It is obviously easier to afford processed products as they are cheap. No matter the effectiveness of a diet, if you can't afford it, it cannot help you at all. Fasting is in the first position of cost-effectiveness since it is completely free. You don't have to purchase any meals, so it costs you no cash. There's no reason for you to purchase costly meals or supplements or any drug that makes it cheap for all.

Simple to practice

Intermediate fasting is easy to do and doesn't have any complicated scheduling, it is quite direct. This causes it to be simpler to pursue and more efficient than many diets.

Opens up your mind

It enables you to regulate your mental procedures as IF opens up your body. You are used to responding to your body's urges because you consume whenever you feel slightly hungry. You are released from the control of your body as a result of practicing IF.

Corrects insulin resistance

This is the simplest and easiest route to reduce insulin resistance and insulin levels. It has a highly effective impact. It works better than a rigid low carb diet.

Improves your metabolism

Intermittent fasting enhances your metabolism by considerably reducing the number of calories you eat in one day. During the feeding time you have, it is almost possible to eat the suggested daily calorific requirements. This causes modifications in the body and fat burning. It also helps you to burn fat, even if you eat the normal calories as your system requires, as it will make you burn fat for power instead of carbs.

Disadvantages of Intermittent Fasting

Getting Started Takes an Adjustment

Any lifestyle change takes an adjustment, and it can take months for something to become a habit. Naturally, intermittent fasting is quite an adjustment for people who are used to grazing on food throughout the day. This means that if you push yourself to go into an advanced version of intermittent fasting when you first begin, you can become overwhelmed. But if you start slowly and allow your body to adjust in its own time, you will find it happens much more naturally and becomes easy to stick to.

Potential to Overeat

While intermittent fasting should naturally reduce caloric intake, if a person pushes themselves to fast when they are overly hungry, it might lead to overeating during their eating window. This is because the person feels hungry for so long when fasting when they can finally eat their body believes it must make up for the calories it missed. The result is that the person either hits a weight loss plateau or even experience increased weight.

Possible Leptin Imbalance

The hormone leptin is important as it signals to your body that you are full have no longer need to eat. But when a person practices intermittent fasting, it may temporarily disrupt this hormone's production. However, this is usually only a short-term problem, and once a person's body adjusts to their fasting and eating windows, their leptin will balance itself out. Typically, a leptin imbalance is only a real problem when a person dives head-first into intermittent fasting and attempt to practice advanced level fasting when they are still only a beginner.

You May Become Dehydrated

Many people do not drink enough water. In general, doctors recommend that we drink half of our body's weight in pounds in ounces of water.

Not only do many people not drink enough water as it is, but this can make dehydration worse when a person is practicing fasting. This is because fasting boosts the metabolism, and when your cells are in a metabolic accelerated state, they require more water for fuel. If you are not giving them enough water during periods of fasting, you can quickly become dehydrated. Not only that but when fasting, you are likely to lose a lot of water weight, which can result in dehydration and a deficiency in electrolytes. Make sure that you not only drink plenty of water but also consume enough electrolytes to prevent this. Thankfully, dehydration is easy to avoid if you remain proactive.

Not Everyone Can Practice Intermittent Fasting

Intermittent fasting is a beautiful and healthy lifestyle for the general population. After all, the human body is designed for practice periods of fasting naturally. However, not every person can practice fasting. Some people, due to chronic illness, may be unable to participate. Ultimately, you must ask your doctor if you are healthy enough to practice short-term fasting.

It can trigger the re-feeding syndrome

This is a hazardous and fatal disorder that can happen if you suffer from malnutrition. It is when electrolyte and liquid imbalances occur when malnourished individuals have been hospitalized for a long time and eat again after a long time. The chance of acquiring re-feeding syndrome increases when bodily weight is very small and not eating for more than ten days.

Having low energy.

Although after a while starvation passes, life isn't predictable. You can take part in a tiresome activity that makes you hungry and ultimately unproductive until the hunger goes or you eat. You may have been used to eating a bunch of snacks during the day and quit instantly due to fasting, which may cause a few side-effects. These side effects involve headaches, bad temper, and lack of power, constipation and low levels of concentration. It may also decrease your motivation. This sort of fasting can have an adverse fitness effect if you have a health condition. It is not suitable for all. For example, hypoglycemic people require glucose all day, so they can't profit from fasting.

Interfere with the social side of eating

Eating from ancient times was a significant social event. Special times, festivities, milestone accomplishment and other activities require meal sharing with your friends. IF can mess with your personal life when you change your routine which may not correspond to the regular eating schedule. During occasions where everyone eats and eats, you may stand out as the one who does not want to participate. Many activities including dinner meetings, family meals, and romantic meals are missed among many others.

Reproductive complications in some women

If the fasting is carried out in a fashion that mainly restricts carbs and protein, it can trigger fertility problems in females, lead to electrolyte defects and trigger nutritional deficits. There are also long-term adverse health effects. Intermediate fasting is linked to menstrual, premature menopause and health problems. Research indicates that ovary size can be reduced, thus influencing reproduction, in addition to decreasing bodily volume.

Digestive complications

It can lead to problems linked to digestion. When food is eaten too rapidly, a large meal may cause digestive problems. People who tend to have larger dishes during the feeding period, require to digest them for a longer period of time. It increases the pressure on your digestive system, triggering indigestion and bloating. This will have a stronger impact on people with weak guts.

Weight regains

Intermittent acceleration reduces the body's reliance on carbohydrates for fuel and decreases fat dependency for power. There is an improvement in the decomposition of stored fats. The body undergoes physiological changes as a reaction to a drastic decrease in the body's power consumption. Simply put, this implies that you may not be able to keep your weight or even gain more weight despite extreme dietary restrictions.

Having seen the strengths and downsides of this fasting protocol, it is evident that the amount and weight of each benefit is more advantageous than the downsides. Intermittent fasting will greatly improve the quality and the quantity of your life without a doubt.

Chapter 7

Best Exercises For Women Over 50/What to Eat Before Your Exercises

Physical activity is the last piece of the weight loss triad, but it is in no way less important. Exercising gets your blood pumping, releases endorphins after and during workouts, and may help you burn extra calories. The number of calories you burn will depend on the type of exercise, the duration, and intensity. However, this is generally a small amount and is nowhere near the number of calories you burn from the basal metabolic rate. Instead, exercise helps in other ways. In the case of intermittent fasting, it can help regulate your energy levels and deplete available glycogen stores, forcing your body to burn fat if it isn't already. Remember those old school workout videos with everyone talking about "feeling the burn?" Very rarely will exercise directly burn fat. In fact, fat only gets burned after glycogen stores are gone (which takes a while). Most amateur athletes never get to that level of performance. We sometimes hear that burning x amounts of calories (3,500, for example) equals burning 1 pound of fat. More specifically, you are burning 3,500 calories, which results in losing one pound of fat, more or less.

Many people feel that exercising on an empty stomach is bad for you. One way this could be true is by causing a significant drop in blood sugar levels. Here, diabetics need to be extra careful. The best time for them to exercise would be just hours after starting a fast—when food energy is still running high in the body. An exercise of any kind will naturally bring blood sugar levels down. If someone can't regulate blood sugar levels efficiently (diabetes) they run the danger of having a serious episode of low blood sugar. Otherwise, the body can detect that blood sugar levels are dropping and make an adequate response to metabolize glycogen. People who find it difficult to exercise while fasting may elect to "cheat" by having a small meal prior to the workout. Protein shakes are notorious for this, as they tend to be high in both carbohydrates and proteins. Mixing whey protein with water may run anywhere between 120 and 400 calories depending on how much powder is used. Mixing it with milk will increase the calorie content significantly. But normally protein shakes aren't required to get through exercise.

If you are already acclimatized to the fat burning stage of a low-carb diet, you will find it easier to get through regular exercise even when fasted. Trying to get a full workout in during the first week of Keto will prove difficult. Trying to exercise in the middle of a fast is also hard because you will suffer from the symptoms of low blood sugar. Diabetics will need to take precautions against them. Since a diabetic should be monitoring blood sugar levels regularly, they should schedule a blood meter test shortly before deciding to exercise. If their blood sugar is too low, they simply shouldn't do the workout. At the very least, they should eat something to get these levels back to a range that is healthy for physical activity. Like with fasting, the workout should be terminated if you experience any symptoms of increased dizziness, lightheadedness, vomiting, or loss of consciousness.

The types of exercise you decide on undertaking will depend on your fitness goals. A good general recommendation for people who wish to be healthier is resistance training at least twice a week alongside the recommended 150 minutes a week of moderate to intense aerobic activity. These 150 minutes can further be increased to 300 minutes to receive even more benefits. These include lowering the risk of cardiovascular disease, reduction of the risk of cancers, and a greater increase in weight-loss potential from physical activity alone. Whether a full 300 minutes of exercise is sustainable a week while fasting will depend on the fitness level of the person, as well as what their fasting routines look like—for example, somebody who is doing the "5:2" Method may simply decide not to exercise on their fasting days. Others who fast daily by skipping breakfast (and fasting overnight) may decide to get the workout done after the fasting period is over. Breaking the fast with a small meal and then doing the workout afterward is a good option. Exercise gets a little trickier on those longer (1–3 days or more) fasts. The considerations are still the same and the risk of a low blood sugar episode increases.

Aerobic Exercise

Anything that gets you on your feet and moving around is considered aerobic. In specific, it deals with raising your heart rate for extended periods of time. It comes from the word that means "with oxygen," causing you to breathe faster than usual while giving your body enough oxygen to flow in the blood. Walking, jogging, jump rope, cycling, stair climbing, and countless sports all qualify for aerobic exercise. Current American physical activity guidelines recommend at least 150 minutes of this type of exercise a week. One of the easiest things you can do is walk. Walking is virtually free in most cases and can be a pleasant change of pace. You can take your dog or a buddy along with you to keep you company. These are also called endurance activities because you should be able to maintain them for at least ten minutes at a time. This key here is to get your heart working faster and your breathing to be deeper. You should be working hard but still able to carry on a conversation. These activities will strengthen your heart and lungs which are, after all, very important muscles in your body.

Aerobic exercise while fasted will use glycogen primarily as fuel, depending on how far into the fast you are. If you exercise just after your last meal, you can get an energy boost from that. Believe it or not, people who work out on their fasting period report higher levels of energy that they do during non-fasted workouts. This has primarily to do with the body's secretion HGH, among other things to compensate for the lack of readily available energy. But these levels of energy are usually reserved for people who are used to fasting. If you try to exercise during your first weeks of trying it out, expect major resistance from your body. It is prudent to take things slow and to increase the intensity or duration of fasted workouts gradually. In the meantime, you can exercise on non-fasting days as usual. The purpose here is to engage in some activity that gets your heart pumping faster and your lungs expanding further. Swimming, walking, running, cycling, aerobics classes, dancing – all of these are great activities for getting the circulation going again. Just remember to begin slowly and pay attention to your body. In other words, if something hurts, stop. But make sure it is really hurt. There is a difference between 'Wow I'm really out of shape because I haven't walked anywhere in a while' and 'My knee really hurts when I do that'. And any time you are ever in doubt seek medical attention.

10 emotional tips

Acknowledge your emotional triggers

Leave cellphone at home

Immerse yourself in a new culture

Acknowledge what people are saying

Develop your perspective

Invent yourself

Practice empathy.

Strive for balance.

Get Enough Sleep to Maintain Energy and Increase Productivity

Eat well

Chapter 8

Ketogenic Diet: What It Is, How It Works and How Many Pounds You Can Lose

The ketogenic diet is a nutritional strategy based on reducing carbohydrates in the diet and "requiring" the body to produce glucose it needs to survive and increase the consumption of fat energy in adipose tissue. Effective, very popular, but also controversial: You can lose a lot of weight through the ketogenic diet, but it is not suitable for everyone.

How does it work? This diet is based on the induction of ketosis, a biochemical condition in which the body starts burning "excess" fat after consuming all available sugars. Based on this principle, the ketogenic diet is very effective, but that does not mean it is for everyone and allows you to do it yourself. First, because the underlying mechanism is very subtle and has various parameters that also affect our health.

The state of ketosis, in which the body burns stored fat without sugar, is not easily achieved, let alone maintained. First, it is important to eliminate sources of carbohydrates from everyday foods such as bread, pasta, potatoes and sugar-based products, but also dairy products, nuts, fruits and vegetables, orange and red. The ketogenic diet means "diet that produces the body of ketones" (metabolic residues from energy production).

In the ketogenic diet, ketone bodies are regularly produced in minimal quantities and can be easily disposed of by ventilation of urine and lungs. They reach higher than normal values. The unwanted excess of the ketone body, which is responsible for the tendency to lower blood pH, is called ketosis. Motor activity also has a positive or negative effect (depending on the case) on the status of ketoacidosis. The presence of ketone bodies in blood has various effects on the body; some are considered useful in the slimming process, others are "collateral".

There is no single type of ketogenic diet and all food styles that provide less than necessary calories, carbohydrates and sometimes proteins are ketogenic; they are certainly low carb and potentially ketogenic, for example, the Atkins diet and LCHF (low carb, high fat - low carbohydrate, high fat). Some types of ketogenic diet are used in clinical setting (for example against non-responsive epilepsy, serious obesity associated with certain metabolic pathologies etc.), but these are systems mainly exploited in fitness and also in aesthetic culture.

The ketogenic diet is a nutritional strategy based on the reduction of food carbohydrates, which "obliges" body to independently produce glucose necessary for survival and to increase the energy consumption of the fats contained in the adipose tissue. Regularly produced in minimal quantities, and easily disposable with urine and lung ventilation, in the ketogenic diet the ketone bodies reach a level higher than the normal condition. The unwanted excess of ketone bodies, responsible for the tendency to lower blood pH, is called ketosis.

What to eat in the ketogenic diet?

The most important aspect to reaching the state of ketosis is to eat foods that do not contain carbohydrates, limit those that make few and avoid foods that are rich in them. Recommended foods are:

- ●Meat, fishery products and eggs - the basic group of foods
- ●Cheeses - The fundamental group of foods
- ●Seasoning oils, fats - V fundamental group of foods
- ●Vegetables, greens - VI and VII fundamental group of foods.

The foods not recommended instead, are:

- ●Cereals, potatoes and derivatives - III fundamental group of foods
- ●Legumes - IV fundamental group of foods
- ●Fruits - VI and VII fundamental group of foods
- ●Sweet drinks, various sweets, beer etc.
- ●Generally, it is recommended to maintain a carbohydrate intake of less than or equal to 50 g / day, ideally organized in 3 portions with 20 g each.

A rather strict guideline for a correct ketogenic diet provides for an energy distribution of:

- ●10% from carbohydrates
- ●15-25% of proteins (not forgetting that proteins, also containing glucogenic amino acids, participate in supporting the blood glucose level)

- ●70% or more from fat.

How to understand that you are in ketosis?

To identify a possible state of ketosis it is possible to carry out tests of urine (with special strips for urine), blood (blood ketone meters) or breath (analyzer of ketones in the breath). However, you can also rely on certain "telltale" symptoms, which require no testing:

- ●Dry mouth and feeling thirsty

- ●Increased diuresis (for the filtration of acetoacetate)

- ●Acetonic breath or sweat (due to presence of acetone) that escapes through our breath

- ●Reduction of appetite

- ●Fatigue.

How many ketones must be present in the blood?

There is no real distinction between ketosis and non-ketosis. The level of these compounds is influenced by diet and lifestyle. However, it is possible to affirm that there is an optimal range for the correct functioning of the ketogenic diet:

- ●Below 0.5 mmol of ketones per liter of blood it is not considered ketosis.

- ●Between 0.5-1.5 mmol / l we speak of light ketosis

- ●With 1.5-3 mmol / l ketosis is defined optimal

- ●Values of over 3 mmol / l, in addition to not being more effective, compromise the state of health (especially in case of type 1 diabetes mellitus)

- - •Values above 8-10 mmol / l are difficult to achieve with the diet. Sometimes they are obtained in diseases or through inadequate physical activity; they also relate to very serious symptoms.

How does the ketogenic diet work?

The functioning mechanism of the ketogenic diet is based on the reduction of calories and food carbohydrates which, in association with a correct level of proteins and a high percentage of fat, should improve lipolysis and cellular lipid oxidation, therefore total consumption of fats optimizing weight loss. The production of ketone bodies, which must be absolutely controlled, has the function of moderating the appetite stimulus - for their anorectic effect. Cellular energy production occurs thanks to the metabolization of some substrates, especially glucose and fatty acids. Mostly, this process begins in the cytoplasm (anaerobic glycolysis - without oxygen) and ends in the mitochondria (Krebs cycle, with oxygen and ATP refill).

Note: muscle cells are also capable of oxidizing good quantities of branched chain amino acids. However, two fundamental aspects must be underlined: some tissues, such as the nervous one, function almost exclusively on glucose. The correct cellular use of fatty acids is subject to the presence of glucose which, if deficient, is produced by the liver by neoglucogenesis (starting from substrates such as glucogenic amino acids and glycerol).

Note: Neoglucogenesis alone is not able to definitively satisfy the metabolic demands of the whole organism in the long term. This is why carbohydrates, although they cannot be defined essential, must be considered as essential nutrients.

Residual ketone bodies

During energy production, fatty acids are first reduced to CoA (coenzyme A) and, immediately afterwards, allowed to enter the Krebs cycle. Here they bind to oxaloacetate to achieve further oxidation, ending with the release of carbon dioxide and water. When the production of acetyl CoA by lipolysis exceeds the absorption capacity of oxaloacetate, the formation of so-called ketone bodies takes place.

Note: each ketone body is made up of two acetyl CoA molecules. Ketone bodies are of three types: acetone, acetoacetate and 3-hydroxybutyrate.

Disposal of ketone bodies

Ketone bodies can be further oxidized, in particular by muscle cells, the heart and to a lesser extent by the brain (which mainly uses them in the absence of glucose), or eliminated in the urine and with lung ventilation. Needless to say, increasing the ketone bodies in the blood also increases the workload of the kidneys. If the production of ketone bodies exceeds the body's disposal capacity, they accumulate in the blood giving rise to the so-called ketosis.

Application of the ketogenic diet

This food strategy is mainly used in three contexts (very different from each other):

- ●Weight loss (preferably under medical supervision). Food therapy of certain metabolic pathologies such as chronic hyperglycemia, hypertriglyceridemia (only under medical supervision), high blood pressure and metabolic syndrome (never in the presence of pathologies or suffering of liver and / or kidneys).

- ●Reduction of symptoms associated with childhood epilepsy (only when the subject does not respond to drug therapy and only under medical supervision).

Advantages of the ketogenic diet

The ketogenic diet has many advantages, facilitates weight loss thanks to:

- ●Reduction of total calories;
- ●Maintaining constant blood sugar and insulin levels;
- ●Increased fat consumption for energy purposes;
- ●Increased calorie expenditure - due to "metabolic work";
- ●It has an anorectic effect;
- ●It can be useful in countering the symptoms of epilepsy that does not respond to drugs, especially in children.

Disadvantages of the ketogenic diet

The ketogenic diet can also show several disadvantages, most of which depend on the levels of ketone bodies in the blood:

- ●Increased renal filtration and diuresis (excretion of ketone bodies and nitrogen waste);
- ●Tendency to dehydration;
- ●Increased kidney workload;
- ●Possible toxic effect on the kidneys by ketone bodies;
- ●Possible hypoglycaemia;
- ●Possible hypotension;

It can be particularly harmful for:

- ●Malnourished subjects such as, for example, those affected by eating disorders (DCA).

- ●Type I diabetes.

- ●Pregnant and nurse.

- ●Those who already suffer from liver and / or kidney diseases.

From a therapeutic perspective, if carbohydrates are relevant factors in promoting mortality, not only the reduction of total intake, but also the inhibition of carbohydrate absorption and metabolism should prolong the life span. Finally, it is essential to drink a lot of water: at least two liters per day. This diet - as we have already pointed out - is particularly controversial and over the years has stimulated heated debates among experts. First of all because it basically eliminates many foods from the table, secondly because it does not admit any errors.

In fact, the state of ketosis can only be maintained if all the rules are followed to the letter. Even a single candy or a drink, I can put the biochemical balance at risk, pushing the body to stop burning fat. Not only that: maintaining the weight achieved is very difficult, so once the diet is finished (to be followed with the help of a professional) it will be necessary to reintroduce the foods very gradually. If followed correctly and always under the supervision of a doctor, the ketogenic diet can be useful for eliminating extra pounds without affecting the lean muscle mass. It can also help you achieve excellent goals in a short time, winning where all the diets have failed previously.

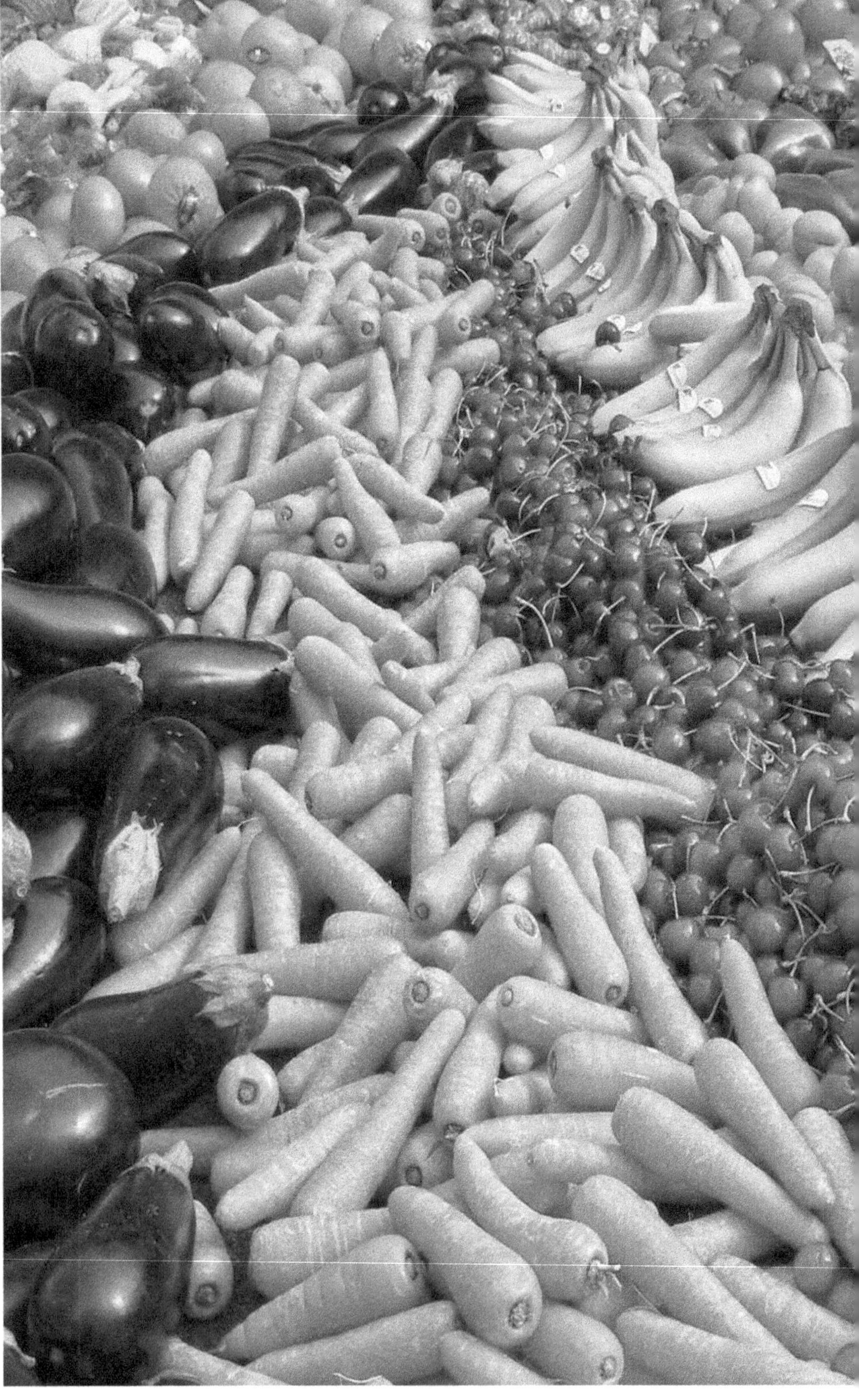

Who can do it and who can not

Dedicated to those in a hurry to make peace with the scale, it promises to lose weight quickly: it is based on the rule of 16 hours of fasting and 8 hours in which 3 meals are allowed, pushes to burn fat and limits the sense of hunger, but it is not suitable for everyone. Like all "extreme" diets, it must always be followed with due care, and absolutely avoided if you are not in perfect health.

In addition to the usual restrictions for pregnant or nursing women, adults, or people with complete pathology, this regimen is not recommended for people who have or have had eating disorders. The risk is to promote a certain lack of education not only for the moment, but also for the right dose of nutrition to consume. Calorie restriction should not cause nutritional deficiencies. It is important to know that anxiety, increased fatigue, and swelling can occur. Behind an inch with a smaller waist is a metabolic revolution and hormone balancing. It is a good idea to know this before you start a new diet, which should always be kept under medical supervision.

Is breakfast the most important meal? Apparently not. You may not know it, but this myth has been denied (I speak of it here). Okay, but is it true that eating small, frequent meals increases your metabolism? No, that's not true either (I'm talking about it here). While these myths have been dispelled, and it has been found that for some they are reliable, for others not, more and more people are interested in intermittent fasting as a method of weight loss, or in a practice known as "meal timing".

Is breakfast the most important meal? Apparently not. You may not know it, but this myth has been denied (I speak of it here). Okay, but is it true that eating small, frequent meals increases your metabolism? No, that's not true either (I'm talking about it here). While these myths have been dispelled, and it has been found that for some they are reliable, for others not, more and more people are interested in intermittent fasting as a method of weight loss, or in a practice known as "meal timing".

In fact, following intermittent fasting does not mean fasting, but reduce the amount of food, often within a span of time that can be 12 hours, 8 hours, 16 hours, and even 4 hours. You eat one or two meals or how much food you want during that period. For example, if I choose to fast 16 hours, my mealtime is 8 hours. In short: there are people who eat once or twice a day and don't eat the rest of their time. According to some, we have seen:

- ●Promotes insulin sensitivity, therefore would adjust blood sugar, sense of satiety, and reduce hunger for sweets;

- ●Improves some health parameters, including cholesterol and triglycerides.

There are people who lose more weight with this diet compared to traditional diets with all three meals. Although this trend is developing, especially among athletes, it is not true that routine fasting is for everyone, and it is not true that you lose more than a normal low calorie diet. However, experts in this study explain that weekly energy balance is important.

So you can eat once a day or ten times: if you eat 1500 calories and need 2000 calories and do it in a week, you have to lose half a pound in the end. Why do some people lose weight through fasting regularly? Just because it's more comfortable to follow them. For people who don't eat breakfast, rest 16 hours and eat 8, or one of 18 and eat 6 hours, that's obviously easy. In short, this helps improve health parameters. But the reality is that if we no longer have to listen to those who say that breakfast is the most important diet, we should not even listen to those who believe that regular fasting is a way to lose weight. To find out if it's right for you, avoid dinner or breakfast by trying to eat within 8 hours. Then weigh at the weekend. If you lose weight and aren't hungry, routine fasting is the right diet for you.

Chapter 9

Benefits of Intermittent Fasting

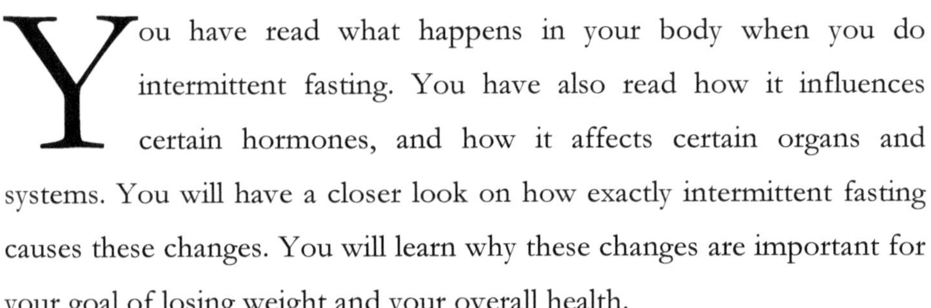

You have read what happens in your body when you do intermittent fasting. You have also read how it influences certain hormones, and how it affects certain organs and systems. You will have a closer look on how exactly intermittent fasting causes these changes. You will learn why these changes are important for your goal of losing weight and your overall health.

Weight Loss

To lose weight, you have to consume consistently fewer calories than how much your body needs. This lower calorie consumption results in a calorie deficit that forces your body to turn to an energy source other than glucose. At first, it will burn glycogen. When this runs out, it will start burning the body fat that we are aiming to lose.

The common approach to induce a caloric deficit is by following a calorie-restricted diet. However, this would require you the tedious work of counting the calories of your every meal, which is impractical, especially if you are eating out. And, with our caloric requirements varying for every single day, your calorie deficit would rarely be consistent.

This is where intermittent fasting can make weight loss easier for you. All you would have to do is follow a schedule for when you can and cannot eat. This would naturally make you lose some meals for the day, which puts your body at a calorie deficit.

Out of the two methods, intermittent fasting is easier to do. And, with one study stating that both methods can provide similar weight loss results, you are basically getting the same benefit for less work with intermittent fasting.

However, fasting provides even more weight loss benefits than simple fat loss. Intermittent fasting also increases the insulin sensitivity, human growth hormone production in your body. These help your body even further in losing unwanted weight from body fat. Here's how these help you in achieving weight loss:

Less body fat stored

Every fasting phase while intermittently fasting depletes the glucose present in your blood and the glycogen stored in your muscles. This helps the body get used to requiring less than its usual insulin levels to respond to increased blood sugar levels. This decreased requirement for insulin means that the body has regained its sensitivity for the hormone.

The increased insulin sensitivity makes the body more efficient in using glucose for energy. With less insulin going around, your blood sugar goes to where it is needed. It would not go to your body fat cells, which will make you regain the weight you lose while fasting or exercising.

Better muscle growth

Fasting increases your body's production of human growth hormone. By itself, an increased production of this hormone does not have any effect on weight loss. But, when it's combined with calorie restriction, a higher production of human growth hormone can accelerate weight loss by helping you burn fat. The increase in fat burning occurs due to human growth hormone increasing the breakdown and use of fat for fueling the body's metabolism.

Do not worry about looking bulky. Women naturally have lower testosterone levels. Because of this, your muscles do not grow in the same way or rate as men. Of course, there are women that choose to bulk up in such a way. However, these are often achieved with external intervention to boost testosterone production.

Maintain lean muscle mass

The problem with most weight loss and fat loss diets is that losing weight comes with losing muscle mass. Losing your muscle mass is the last thing you want when losing weight. It decreases how much calories your body needs on a daily basis. With reduced calorie needs, your body would eventually reach a caloric surplus even if you maintain your caloric intake. This risk of caloric surplus becomes even greater once you achieved your weight loss goal and stop restricting your diet. Either way, you would eventually gain the fat that you lost.

In intermittent fasting, this rebound is not likely to happen since it can preserve your lean muscle mass even when the body is deficient of calories. One study has observed that intermittent fasting can maintain lean muscle mass while promoting fat loss among obese individuals. This helps your body maintain its metabolism while getting rid of unwanted body fat. Because of this, you would not reach a caloric surplus even as long as you maintain your caloric intake.

Maintaining this lean muscle mass is crucial if you aim to have a defined figure when you finally shed the unwanted body fat from your physique. Doing intermittent fasting instead of focusing on restricting calories for weight loss will help you avoid getting the flat muscle look most women get that result from such diets. Of course, maintaining this definition when you achieve your intended fat loss requires that you already have created a foundation of muscle mass for it or working towards it. If you are working towards it while intermittently fasting, you would have to do resistance training.

Improves keto-adaptation

Our bodies normally use both glucose and fat as energy sources. However, due to a diet of high carbohydrates being the norm, we lost the ability to easily switch between using glucose and fat for fueling our metabolism.

Intermittent fasting helps you regain this ability by frequently depleting your body's glucose and stored glycogen. Once this is depleted, the body has no choice but to resort to a fat burning state. Eventually, the body will have an easier time to keto-adapt, which is its ability to switch from glucose to fat for energy.

Better keto-adaptation gives you more stable energy levels so you would have less cravings for food. Also, since your body switches to using fat more quickly, you are burning fat even when the body is only at standing or sitting down.

Decreased food cravings

Normally, when you think that you're hungry, you are actually just craving for food. These instances of food craving are brought about by the rapid or prolonged increase of your insulin levels. Intermittent fasting helps your body learn what it actually means to be hungry by helping it regain its insulin sensitivity. Once it reaches healthy levels of insulin sensitivity, the body stops producing more insulin than it actually needs. As a result, you are less likely to have sugar cravings despite having normal blood sugar levels.

Intermittent fasting also decreases food cravings and increases your tolerance against hunger. It also improves the response of the body when releasing the hormone inducing the sensation of fullness and satiety. As a result, one is less likely to overeat since they can immediately feel when they have eaten enough.

This greatly benefits women doing an intermittent fast. This is due to women being more likely to experience food cravings on a daily basis. To make it worse, food cravings experienced by women are for sweet foods like pastries, chocolate, and ice cream. The increased insulin sensitivity, improved hunger tolerance, and more responsive satiety can help manage these cravings, especially during the culmination of your monthly menstrual cycle when these cravings are at their strongest.

More manageable appetite

Intermittent fasting lowers your appetite. This results to you eating less and helping you maintain or lose weight. This decreased appetite arises from the effect of intermittent fasting on the hormones that regulate your hunger and satiety.

The body decreases its production of leptin and ghrelin after going through a schedule of intermittent fasting. This helps you have more manageable meals than a simple calorie restricted diet. You are essentially eating less since you do not feel like eating more and already feel satisfied with what you ate.

Promotes muscle gain and fat loss at the same time

An intermittent fasting regimen provides the best conditions to make it possible for you to gain muscle and lose fat at the same time. Training during the fasting phase helps your body to use more of its fat stores for energy. Then, when you break your fast after your workout, your body gets the nutrients it needs for recovery and building new muscle proteins. This was what has been observed in a study involving recreationally active individuals following an eight-week schedule of intermittent fasting and resistance training.

Furthermore, intermittent fasting increases your body's production of human growth hormone. Human growth hormone stimulates the various tissues in your body to release IGF-1. IGF-1 promotes amino acid uptake and its synthesis of muscle fibers. As a result, your body gets to recover and adapt to the stresses placed upon it by your workout.

It should be noted that the benefit of losing fat while gaining muscle requires more than following an intermittent fasting regimen. The same rules still apply when it comes to gaining muscle: you need to progressively train your strength and have a diet that supports its growth. You would also have to be smart about your choices for carbohydrates and caloric intake if you also want to lose fat.

Improved recovery from workout

Due to increased insulin sensitivity, your body is more efficient in allocating glucose to where it is needed. This means your muscles get the energy needed to recover from your workout. This energy can be used in helping the muscles recover and grow new muscle proteins.

However, it should be noted that muscle gain can suffer if the body is not getting what it needs from its diet. You have to consume enough calories to provide the energy needed to build muscles. You should also consume enough branch chain amino acids so your body has the necessary building blocks for muscle growth.

Also, with fasting inducing autophagy, your body becomes better at recovery and building muscle. This is due to autophagy improving the efficiency of the cells involved in repairing muscle cells and creating new muscle proteins. The more efficient cells can also help those who experienced muscle damage and trauma since autophagy also improves regeneration of muscle tissues.

An easier method to improve conditions of obesity

Other than problems with a person's genetic make-up, obesity is caused by a lifestyle of low physical activity and high carbohydrate and fat consumption. Those that find themselves in such a situation would usually resort to restricting their calories to lose weight. Unfortunately, most obese individuals often find this approach a drastic approach since the caloric restrictions are far below than what they are used to.

This is where some researchers turned to intermittent fasting as an alternative to help obese women ranging from 35 to 70 years of age. According to the study, intermittent fasting is effective in weight loss even without restricting food intake. The weight loss recorded is an average of 5 percent of their starting weight. Furthermore, if combined with a diet restricting food intake to 70 percent, participants lost twice the weight lost by intermittent fasters that have no dietary restrictions.

It should be noted that doing an intermittent fast without restricting the diet is only good for the short term. It can increase one's fasting insulin levels, which can be detrimental to long-term weight loss goals. This approach is useful as a starting point so obese individuals can gradually reduce their food intake.

Reduces visceral fat

Visceral fat is a body fat type found in your abdominal cavity. It can be found near, attached to, or surrounding your stomach, liver, arteries, and intestines. Unlike subcutaneous fat (the one you find under your skin), visceral fat increase your likelihood for serious health disorders like Alzheimer's disease, type 2 diabetes, liver insulin resistance, colorectal cancer, and breast cancer. Also, this fat increases the inflammation in your body, which could promote the accumulation of plaque in the arteries. Eventually, it could lead to a heart attack, ruptured or blocked arteries, and stroke.

Intermittent fasting can reduce the existing visceral fat in your body in two ways. First, it restricts caloric intake by having a limited time for eating. This helps your body burn body fat – both subcutaneous and visceral. Over time, the body metabolizes visceral fat tissue deposits until these are reduced to harmless amounts.

Second, intermittent fasting induces autophagy in the body. The body's self-eating mechanism protects the body from the formation of these harmful fat deposits. This helps manage and prevent new visceral fat deposits from forming as you are losing the existing ones. As for the existing fat deposits, autophagy increases the rate the body metabolizes visceral fat tissue into energy.

Lower risk for Type 2 Diabetes

Type 2 diabetes is a complication brought about by chronically elevated insulin levels. This causes the body to resist the effects of the hormone. With glucose unregulated, it can easily accumulate in your bloodstream. At its initial stages, the symptoms include increased hunger and thirst, frequent urination, sugar in the urine, blurred vision, and headache. In the long term, it could lead to complications in the cardiovascular system, nervous system, kidneys, eyes, bones, and joints.

Intermittent fasting helps to manage the blood sugar levels by restricting food intake at a set timeframe. The body does not get a new supply of blood sugar while it is restricted from eating. This forces the body to use up the glucose available in its bloodstream. This causes a decline in blood sugar levels. The body detects this decrease and lowers the insulin in its bloodstream.

Furthermore, there is an increase in insulin sensitivity every time a fast ends due to the release of glucagon-like peptide 1 (GLP1). This increased insulin sensitivity frequently occurs with intermittent fasting. In the long run, the body returns its insulin sensitivity to healthy levels.

Aside from this, intermittent fasting improves the overall function of the pancreas. Poor pancreas function is one of the factors believed to worsen conditions of type 2 diabetes (61). This reduced function is caused by pancreatic fat, malfunctioning pancreatic beta cells, or both. With intermittent fasting, these fat deposits in the pancreas are metabolized by the body for energy.

And, with a fast-induced autophagy, the dysfunctional and damaged organelles in the pancreas are broken down into reusable components.

These are then used to build new organelles that let the pancreatic cells secrete insulin into the bloodstream (62).

Alternate day fasting is the method that works best to lower the risk of type 2 diabetes and improve pancreas function. This method was what research has observed to be effective. In this particular regimen, those that experienced improvement followed a 75 percent energy restriction during their fasting days (63).

Maintains and enhances brain health

Anti-aging benefits

As you age, the nerve cells of your brain go through natural changes. These are evidenced by slower reflexes, increasing difficulty in memory recall, reduced cognition, and slower decision-making as we grow old. Unfortunately, aging can be accelerated by the oxidative stress, toxic exposure, and amyloid beta-accumulation on our brain and its cells.

Intermittent fasting can help slow down these effects caused by aging. In some cases, these effects are even completely reversed. This anti-aging effect arises from the use of ketone bodies as an energy source while the body is under a fasting phase.

The use of ketone bodies causes neurons in your brain's hippocampus to produce more mitochondria for energy production that increases the efficiency of each cell in doing its job.

It increases the expression of the BDNF protein. This results in the inhibition of brain cell death, which helps preserve old brain cells so it can be repaired or reused by the body through autophagy. It also boosts the adaptability of the synapses of brain cells, which helps in its ability to change and adapt to the new information our brain receives or transmits.

Ketone bodies also prevent the production of free radicals in neurons. This is due to free radicals being a by-product of glucose metabolism. In addition to this, ketones stimulate the antioxidant activity present in neurons.

Aside from introducing ketone bodies to the brain, the repeated switching between fat and glucose metabolism boosts the resilience of your brain's cells and its neuronal circuits (64). The shifting strengthens the stress resistance of activated brain cells and increases the preparedness of these cells to transmit signals through the nervous system. This effect seems to be caused by the molecular recycling and pathway repair occurring in the cell due to the autophagy induced by fasting. This is combined with the creation of new neurons, synapses, and mitochondria when the body shifts into growth upon breaking the fast. Due to the nature of intermittent fasting, these two phases occur repeatedly in a cycle. This translates to a compounding effect of increasing efficiency for the existing cells and promoting cell, synapse, and mitochondria growth.

Lastly, when breaking a fast, the body releases the hormone glucagon-like peptide 1 (GLP1). The GLP1 hormone promotes insulin release from the pancreas and increases the insulin sensitivity of various cells. It does this by interacting with the neurons found in your spinal cord and those that connect it to your different organs. This interaction has an added effect of improving the signal cognition, stress resistance, and synaptic plasticity of these nerves. This results in the nerves being more efficient in transmitting signals between your brain and the various organs found in your cardiovascular system and digestive system. Moreover, since it can cross the blood-brain barrier, these benefits are also felt by your brain cells.

Chapter 10

Breakfast Recipes

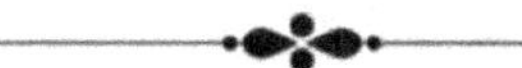

Zucchini Omelet

Preparation time: 4 minutes

Cooking time: 3 hours and 30 minutes

Servings: 6

Ingredients:

1½ cups red onion, chopped

1 tablespoon olive oil

2 garlic cloves, minced

2 teaspoons fresh basil, chopped

6 eggs, whisked

A pinch of sea salt and black pepper

8 cups zucchini, sliced

6 ounces fresh tomatoes, peeled, crushed

Directions

In a bowl, mix all the ingredients except the oil and the basil.

Grease the slow cooker with the oil, spread the omelet mix in the bowl, cover and cook on low for 3 hours and 30 minutes.

Divide the omelet between plates, sprinkle the basil on top and serve for breakfast.

Nutrition:

Calories: 120

Fat: 18g

Protein: 15g

Carbs: 1.8g

Chili Omelet

Preparation time: 5 minutes

Cooking time: 3 hours and 30 minutes

Servings: 4

Ingredients:

2 garlic cloves, minced

1 tablespoon olive oil

1 red bell pepper, chopped

1 small yellow onion, chopped

1 teaspoon chili powder

2 tablespoons tomato puree

½ teaspoon sweet paprika

A pinch of salt and black pepper

1 tablespoon parsley, chopped

4 eggs, whisked

Directions

In a bowl, mix all the ingredients except the oil and the parsley and whisk them well.

Grease the slow cooker with the oil, add the egg mixture, cover and cook on low for 3 hours and 30 minutes.

Divide the omelet between plates, sprinkle the parsley on top and serve for breakfast.

Nutrition:

Calories: 100

Fat: 10g

Protein: 15g

Carbs: 1.8g

Basil and Cherry Tomato Breakfast

Preparation time: 4 minutes

Cooking time: 4 hours

Servings: 4

Ingredients:

1 tablespoon olive oil

2 yellow onions, chopped

2 pounds cherry tomatoes, halved

3 tablespoons tomato puree

2 garlic cloves, minced

A pinch of sea salt and black pepper

1 bunch basil, chopped

Directions

Grease the slow cooker with the oil, add all the ingredients, cover and cook on high for 4 hours.

Stir the mixture, divide it into bowls and serve for breakfast.

Nutrition:

Calories: 90

Fat: 1g

Protein: 1g

Carbs: 1.8g

Carrot Breakfast Salad

Preparation time: 5 minutes

Cooking time: 4 hours

Servings: 4

Ingredients:

2 tablespoons olive oil

2 pounds baby carrots, peeled and halved

3 garlic cloves, minced

2 yellow onions, chopped

½ cup vegetable stock

1/3 cup tomatoes, crushed

A pinch of salt and black pepper

Directions

In your slow cooker, combine all the ingredients, cover and cook on high for 4 hours.

Divide into bowls and serve for breakfast.

Nutrition:

Calories: 50

Fat: 10g

Protein: 10g

Carbs: 1.8g

Garlic Zucchini Mix

Preparation time: 5 minutes

Cooking time: 6 hours

Servings: 6

Ingredients:

4 cups zucchinis, sliced

2 tablespoons olive oil

1 teaspoon Italian seasoning

A pinch of salt and black pepper

1 teaspoon garlic powder

Directions

In your slow cooker, mix all the ingredients, cover and cook on Low for 6 hours.

Divide into bowls and serve for breakfast.

Nutrition:

Calories: 60

Fat: 0.7g

Protein: 1.5g

Carbs: 1.8g

Crustless Broccoli Sun-dried Tomato Quiche

Preparation time: 4 minutes

Cooking time: 3 hours and 30 minutes

Servings: 6

Ingredients:

12.3-ounce box extra-firm tofu drained and dried

1 ½ cup broccoli, chopped

2 teaspoons yellow mustard

1 tablespoon tahini

1 tablespoon cornstarch

¼ cup old fashioned oats

½ teaspoon turmeric

3-4 dashes Tabasco sauce

½-1 teaspoon salt

½ cup artichoke hearts, chopped

2/3 cup tomatoes, sun-dried, soaked in hot water

1/8 cup vegetable broth

Directions

Preheat your oven to 375 degrees Fahrenheit.

Prepare a 9" pie plate or springform pan with parchment paper or cooking spray.

Put all of the leeks and broccoli on a cookie sheet and drizzle with vegetable broth, salt, and pepper. Bake for about 20-30 min.

In the meantime, add the tofu, garlic, nutritional yeast, lemon juice, mustard, tahini, cornstarch, oats, turmeric, salt, and a few dashes of Tabasco in a food processor. When the mixture is smooth, taste for heat and add more Tabasco as needed.

Place cooked vegetables with artichoke hearts and tomatoes in a large bowl. With a spatula, scrape in tofu mixture from the processor. Mix carefully, so all of the vegetables are well distributed. If the mixture seems too dry, add a little vegetable broth or water.

Add mixture to pie plate muffin tins, or springform pan and spread evenly.

Bake for about 35 min. or until lightly browned.

Cool before serving. It is delicious, both warm and chilled!

Nutrition:

Calories: 150

Fat: 18g

Protein: 15g

Carbs: 1.8g

Chocolate Pancakes

Preparation time: 5 minutes

Cooking time: 80 minutes

Servings: 6

Ingredients:

1 ¼ cup gluten-free flour of choice

1 tablespoon ground flaxseed

1 tablespoon baking powder

3 tablespoons nutritional yeast

2 tablespoons unsweetened cocoa powder

¼ teaspoon of sea salt

1 cup unsweetened, unflavored almond milk

1 tablespoon vegan mini chocolate chips (optional)

1 teaspoon vanilla extract

¼ teaspoon stevia powder or 1 tablespoon pure maple syrup

1 tablespoon apple cider vinegar

¼ cup unsweetened applesauce.

Directions

Get a medium bowl and mix all the dry ingredients (flour, baking powder, flaxseed, cocoa powder, yeast, salt, and optional chocolate chips). Whisk until evenly combined.

In a separate small bowl, combine wet ingredients except for the applesauce (almond milk, vanilla extract, apple cider vinegar, maple syrup, or stevia powder).

Add wet ingredient mixture and applesauce to the dry ingredients and mix by hand until ingredients are just combined.

The batter should sit for 10 minutes. It will rise and thicken, possibly doubling in size.

Heat an electric griddle or nonstick skillet to medium heat and spray with a small amount of nonstick spray, if desired. Scoop batter into 3-inch rounds. Much like traditional pancakes, bubbles will start to appear. When bubbles start to burst, flip pancakes and cook for 1-2 minutes. Yields 12 pancakes.

Nutrition:

Calories: 150

Fat: 18g

Protein: 15g

Carbs: 1.8g

Breakfast Scramble

Preparation time: 5 minutes

Cooking time: 60 minutes

Servings: 7

Ingredients:

1 large head cauliflower, cut up

1 seeded, diced green bell pepper

1 seeded, diced red bell pepper

2 cups sliced mushrooms (approximately 8 oz whole mushrooms)

1 peeled, diced red onion

3 peeled, minced cloves of garlic

Sea salt

1 ½ teaspoons turmeric

1–2 tablespoons of low-sodium soy sauce

¼ cup nutritional yeast (optional)

½ teaspoon black pepper

Directions

1. Sauté green and red peppers, mushrooms, and onion in a medium saucepan or skillet over medium-high heat until onion is translucent (should be 7–8 min). Add an occasional tablespoon or two of water to the pan to prevent vegetables from sticking.

2. Add cauliflower and cook until florets are tenders. It should be 5 to 6 minutes.

3. Add, pepper, garlic, soy sauce, turmeric, and yeast (if using) to the pan and cook for about 5 minutes.

Nutrition:

Calories: 180

Fat: 18g

Protein: 15g

Carbs: 1.8g

Oatmeal

Preparation time: 5 minutes

Cooking time: 30 minutes

Servings: 4

Ingredients:

Almond milk, unsweetened, one cup

Flaxseed, whole, one tablespoon

Sunflower seeds, one tablespoon

Chia seeds, one tablespoon

Salt, one half teaspoon

Directions

Dump all of the ingredients together into a small pan and bring the mixture to a boil in a saucepan over medium heat. When it comes to a boil, reduce the heat and allow the mix to simmer gently for two to three minutes until the mix is the desired thickness. Drop a pat of butter on the top and enjoy.

Nutrition:

Calories 621

Net carbs 9 grams

Protein 10 grams

Coconut Cream with Berries

Preparation time: 5 minutes

Cooking time: 30 minutes

Servings: 4 Serves

Ingredients:

Coconut cream, one ha lf cup

Vanilla extract, one teaspoon

Strawberries, fresh, two ounces

Directions

Mix the ingredients together well by using a hand mixer or an immersion mixer if one is available. An added teaspoon of coconut oil will increase the amount of fat in this dish.

Nutrition:

Calories 415

Net carbs9 grams

Fat42 grams

Protein 5 grams

Seafood Omelet

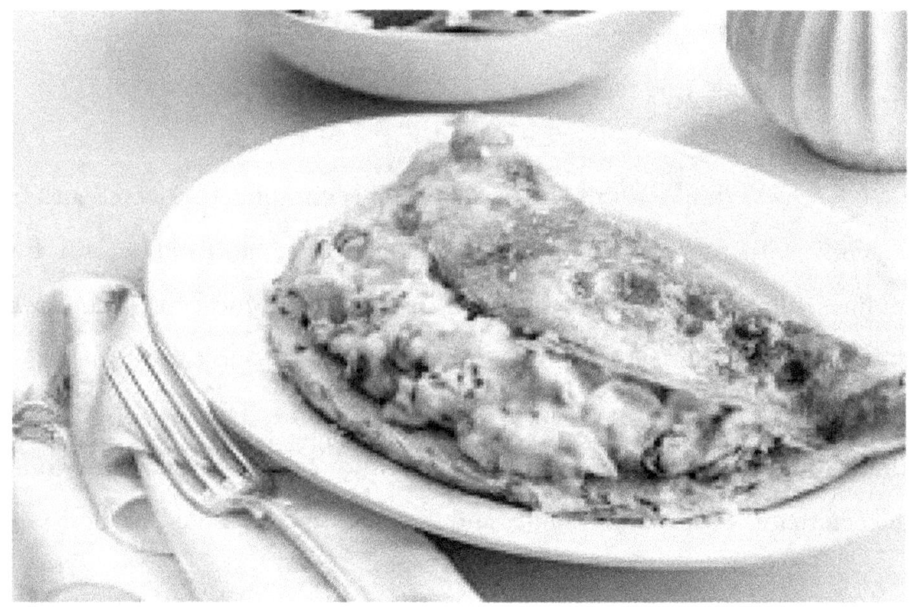

Preparation time: 5 minutes

Cooking time: 30 minutes

Servings: 2

Ingredients:

Shrimp, cooked, five ounces

Eggs, six

Butter, two tablespoons

Olive oil, two tablespoons

Chives, fresh or dried, one tablespoon

Mayonnaise, one half cup

Cumin, ground, one half teaspoon

Thyme, one quarter teaspoon

Garlic, two cloves minced

Red chili pepper, one diced

Salt, one half teaspoon

White pepper, one teaspoon

Directions

Toss the shrimp with the olive oil until it is completely covered and fry it gently with the cumin, garlic, salt, chili pepper, and pepper for five minutes. While the shrimp mix cools beat the eggs and pours them into the skillet. Let the eggs sit undisturbed while they cook until the edges begin to brown and the center has mostly set firm. Then add the chives and the mayonnaise to the shrimp mixture. Pour the shrimp mixture onto the egg that is frying in the skillet and fold the omelet in half, frying for an additional three minutes on each side.

Nutrition:

Calories 872

Net carbs 4 grams

Fat 83 grams

Spinach and Pork with Fried Eggs

Preparation time: 5 minutes

Cooking time: 30 minutes

Servings: 2

Ingredients:

Spinach, baby, two cups

Pork loin, smoked, six ounces cut into chunks

Eggs, four

Salt, one half teaspoon

Black pepper, one teaspoon

Walnuts, chopped, one quarter cup

Cranberries, one quarter cup frozen

Butter, three tablespoons

Directions

Wash, dry, and chop the baby spinach. Fry the spinach in the butter for five minutes stirring continuously. Remove the spinach from the pan and let it drain on a paper towel. Fry the chunks of pork loin in the same skillet for five minutes. Remove the pork from the skillet and then put the cooked baby spinach back in, adding the nuts and cranberries. Stir constantly while this is cooking for five minutes. Pour the mix into a bowl. Fry the eggs and place two on each plate with half of the spinach mixture. Serve with the chunks of fried pork loin.

Nutrition:

Calories 1033

Net carbs 8 grams

Fat 99 grams

Protein 26 grams

Smoked Salmon Sandwich

Preparation time: 5 minutes

Cooking time: 30 minutes

Servings: 2

Ingredients:

TOPPING

Eggs, four

Chives, fresh, chop, one tablespoon

Smoked salmon, three ounces

Heavy whipping cream, two tablespoons

Salt, one half teaspoon

White pepper, one half teaspoon

Kale, one-ounce chop fine

Butter, two tablespoons

Chili powder, one quarter teaspoon

Olive oil, two tablespoons

SPICY PUMPKIN BREAD

Lard, one tablespoon

Pumpkin puree, fourteen ounces

Coconut oil, .25 cup

Eggs, three

Pumpkin seeds, one third cup

Walnuts, chopped, one third cup

Baking powder, one tablespoon

Pumpkin pie spice, two tablespoons

Flaxseed, one half cup

Coconut flour, one and one quarter cups

Almond flour, one and one quarter cups

Psyllium husk powder, ground, two tablespoons

Salt, one teaspoon

Directions

Heat oven to 400. Use the lard to grease a nine by nine pan. Add the baking powder, pumpkin pie spice, nuts, psyllium husk powder, flaxseed, both flours, salt, and seeds into a bowl and mix together well. Use a separate bowl to cream together the oil, pumpkin puree, and egg. Gently pour this mixture into the dry ingredients and fold both together until all of the ingredients are well moistened. Spoon this entire mixture into the greased baking pan and bake it for one hour. Allow the bread to cool completely.

When the bread is done beat together the cream and eggs with the pepper and salt. Scramble the egg mix in the melted butter for five minutes, stirring constantly and then mix in the chili powder. Slice off two slices of the pumpkin bread and place them in the toaster to toast for three minutes. Butter the toasted pumpkin bread and lay each slice on a plate. Top each slice with the kale and the smoked salmon. Place the eggs on top of this and sprinkle with the chives.

Nutrition:

Calories 678

Net carbs 3 grams

Fat 55 grams

Protein 41 grams

Shrimp Deviled Eggs

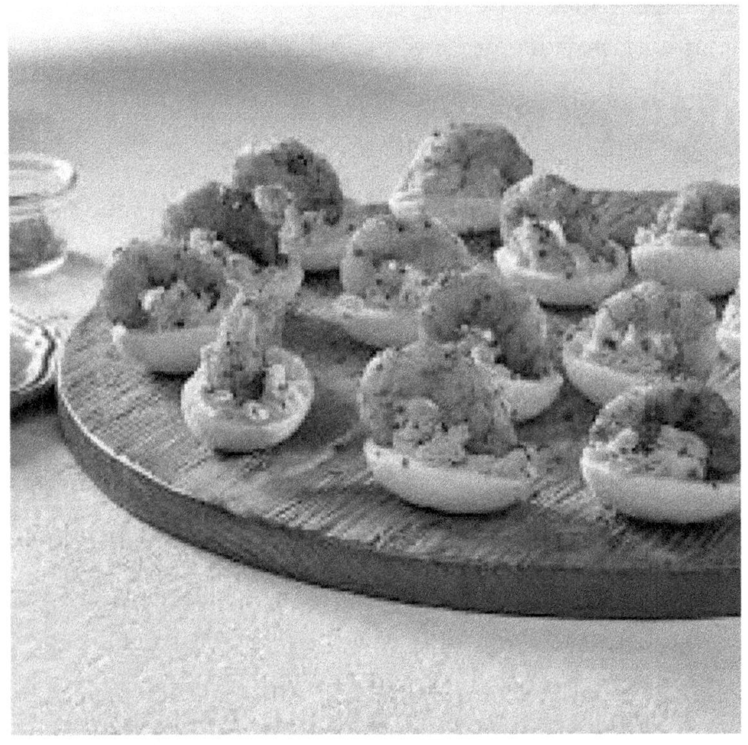

Preparation time: 5 minutes

Cooking time: 30 minutes

Servings: 4

Ingredients:

Chives, chopped, one teaspoon

Mayonnaise, one quarter cup

Eggs, four, hard boiled

Dill sprigs, eight fresh

Tabasco sauce, one teaspoon

Shrimp, peeled and deveined, eight large fully cooked*

Salt, one half teaspoon

White pepper, one half teaspoon

Directions

Carefully peel the chilled hard-boiled eggs and then cut them in half the long way and remove the yolks. Put the yolks into a bowl and use a dinner fork to gently mash the yolks and then add the Tabasco, salt, and mayonnaise. Mix all of this together well and then carefully spoon the mixture back into the egg whites. Top each egg with one cooked shrimp and a sprig of dill.

*Shrimp are sold whole or peeled and deveined. You can peel them yourself and remove the vein but the cost difference to buy them already peeled and deveined (P & D) in very small and worth the price.

Nutrition:

Calories 163

Net carbs 5 grams

Fat 15 grams

Protein 7 grams

Scrambled Eggs with Halloumi Cheese

Preparation time: 5 minutes

Cooking time: 30 minutes

Servings: 2

Ingredients:

Eggs, four

Bacon, four slices

Salt, one half teaspoon

Black pepper, one teaspoon

Chili powder, one quarter teaspoon

Black olives, pitted if needed, one half cup

Parsley, fresh, one half cup chop fine

Scallions, two

Olive oil, two tablespoons

Halloumi cheese, diced from a block, three ounces

Directions

Chop finely the bacon and the cheese. Fry the bacon and the cheese with the scallions in the olive oil for five minutes. While this mixture is frying beat the eggs well with the parsley, pepper, chili powder, and salt. Dump the egg mix onto the bacon cheese mix in the skillet and scramble all together for three minutes while stirring constantly. Add in the olives and cook for three more minutes.

Nutrition:

Calories 667

Carbs 4 grams

Fat 59 grams

Protein 28 grams

Chapter 11

Lunch Recipes

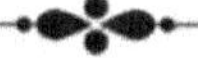

Shrimp Avocado Melt

Preparation Time: 10 minutes

Cooking Time: 5 minutes

Servings: 2

Ingredients

2 ounce shredded cheddar cheese

1 avocado, sliced

2 ounce shredded mozarella cheese

2 tbsp chopped chilies

1 pinch of garlic powder

2 tbsp butter

1 tbsp sesame oil

5 ounce cooked shrimp

Salt and pepper to taste

1/3 cup roasted cashews

2 lettuce leaves

Directions:

Melt the butter in a skillet.

Add the sesame oil to it. Add the garlic and cook until it becomes golden.

Add the cashew nuts, shrimp, chilies and toss for 1 minute.

Add the cheese, salt and pepper and toss until the cheese melts.

Transfer the mixture to a bowl.

Add the avocado slices and mix well.

Spread the mixture onto the lettuce leaves.

Wrap them tightly and seal using a toothpick.

Enjoy.

Nutrition:

Calories: 777

Fat: 63.9 g

Carbs: 23.7g

Protein: 36.1 g

Yellow Squash Soup

Preparation Time: 10 minutes

Cooking Time: 45 minutes

Servings: 6

Ingredients

4 cups chopped yellow squash

1 tbsp olive oil

1 tsp butter

1 onion, chopped

2 eggs

Salt and pepper to taste

½ cup heavy whipping cream

1 cup shredded cheese, divided

2 garlic cloves, mince

1/3 cup roasted chopped almonds

Directions:

Preheat your oven to 400 degrees F.

Add parchment paper onto a baking sheet.

Arrange the squash cubes onto the baking sheet.

Add some oil on top and season using salt.

Bake in the oven for about 30 minutes.

Let it cool down completely and then add to a blender. Blend into a smooth paste.

In a pot whisk the eggs nicely.

Add the squash, garlic, onion, butter, and salt and pepper.

Cook for 5 minutes and add the whipping cream and cheese.

Cook for only 3 minutes.

Serve hot with roasted almonds on top.

Nutrition:

Calories: 228

Fat: 19.6 g

Carbs: 6.7g

Protein: 8.6 g

Meatball Soup

Preparation Time: 1 hour

Cooking Time: 25 minutes

Servings: 6

Ingredients

2 eggs

2 pounds ground chicken or turkey

Salt to taste

1.2 cup soy sauce

4 cups chicken stock

2 garlic cloves, mince

1 tbsp butter

1 tsp ground ginger

Fresh herbs of your choice

Pepper to taste

½ cup sliced onion

1 tsp chopped spring onions

Directions:

In a mixing bowl whisk the eggs finely.

Add the ground chicken or turkey and mix well.

Add the sliced onion, ground ginger, minced garlic and soy sauce.

Mix well and use your hands to create meatballs.

Cover the top of the bowl using a plastic wrap and add to the refrigerator.

Keep it for marinating for 30 minutes or longer.

Take a pot and add the chicken stock.

Add the butter, spring onions, and season using salt and pepper.

Now take out the meatballs and once the stock is at its boiling point, drop them carefully into the pot.

Cover with lid and cook on medium heat for 10 minutes.

Add the fresh herbs and take off the heat.

Serve hot.

Nutrition:

Calories: 90

Fat: 6 g

Carbs: 0.8g

Protein: 7.8 g

Salmon with Spring onion and Sesame Seeds

Preparation Time: 10 minutes

Cooking Time: 20 minutes

Servings: 4

Ingredients

4 salmon fillets

Salt and pepper to taste

1 tsp dried dill weed

1 tbsp soy sauce

2 tsp chopped spring onion

1 tsp sesame seeds

1 tsp onion powder

1 tsp sesame oil

2 tbsp butter

Directions:

Debone the salmon fillets carefully.

Season the fish fillets using salt, pepper, onion powder and dill weed.

Let it marinate for 30 minutes.

In a pan heat the sesame oil over medium heat.

Fry the salmon fillets until they become slightly golden in color.

Transfer onto a plate.

Into the same pan, melt the butter.

Add the sesame seeds and add the spring onion.

Add the soy sauce and cook for 1 minute.

Drizzle the sauce on top of the fillets.

Serve hot.

Nutrition

Calories: 262

Fat: 18.1 g

Carbs: 0.7g

Protein: 22.8 g

Cauliflower Leek Soup

Preparation Time: 10 minutes

Cooking Time: 1 hour

Servings: 8

Ingredients

3 leeks, diced

1 tsp thinly diced ginger

3 garlic cloves

8 cups vegetable broth

3 tbsp butter

2 tbsp olive oil

1 cauliflower heat, chopped

Salt and pepper to taste

1 cup heavy cream

Directions:

Cut off the stem of the leek and cauliflower. Wash them thoroughly.

Chop them into small pieces.

Add to a pressure cooker with broth.

Cover and cook on high heat for 10 minutes.

Use a hand blender to make the mixture perfectly smooth. If you do not have a hand blender, transfer the mixture into a food processor or a blender and then make it smooth.

Now add some oil to a pot.

Fry the garlic and ginger until they are slightly golden.

Return the soup into the pot and mix well.

Add the salt, pepper and heavy cream.

Cook for another 10 minutes.

Serve hot with fresh coriander on top. You can also add some fresh diced ginger on top too.

Nutrition

Calories: 155

Fat: 13.1 g

Carbs: 8.3g

Protein: 2.4 g

Fish Carrot Potato Salad

Preparation Time: 10 minutes

Cooking Time: 20 minutes

Servings: 2

Ingredients

1 fish fillet of your choice

2 carrots

6-10 green beans

Fresh herbs of your choice

2-4 radishes

1 tbsp olive oil

2 small potatoes

2 tbsp butter

1 lemon

1 tbsp honey

Salt to taste

Pepper to taste

Directions:

Discard the bones of the fish. Keep the skin on, it will add flavor to the salad.

In a pan heat the oil over medium high heat.

Add the fish and fry it until it becomes crisp.

Transfer to a plate.

Now peel the carrots, potatoes, radish and cut into thin long sticks.

Cut the potato into wedges. Cut the lemon into wedges. Squeeze out 1 tsp of lemon juice out of them. Leave the rest for garnishing.

In a skillet melt the butter over medium heat.

Slowly fry the potatoes, carrots, green beans and radish.

Assemble the vegetables, the fish onto a serving plate.

Add lemon wedges, fresh herbs on top.

Drizzle the honey and season the salad using salt and pepper.

Nutrition

Calories: 152

Fat: 7.4 g

Carbs: 3.7g

Protein: 23.9 g

Chapter 12

Dinner Recipes

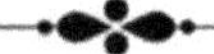

Cheesy Broccoli Soup

Preparation Time: 10 minutes

Cooking Time: 30 minutes

Servings: 6

Ingredients

2 pounds broccoli, chopped

Salt to taste

5 cups vegetable broth

¼ cup shredded cheddar cheese

1 tbsp olive oil

¼ cup lemon juice

2 garlic cloves, mince

1 white onion, chopped

Pepper to taste

Directions:

Heat the olive oil in a pan with medium heat.

Fry the onion for 1 minute and then add the garlic. Fry until the garlic becomes golden in color.

Toss in the broccoli and stir for 3 minutes.

Pour in the vegetable broth.

Add salt, pepper and mix well.

Cook for 20 minutes or until your broccoli is perfectly cooked through.

Take off the heat and let it cool down a bit.

Add to a blender, and blend it until your soup is perfectly smooth.

Transfer the soup into the pot again and heat it over medium heat.

Add lemon juice, cheddar cheese and check if it needs more seasoning.

Serve hot with more cheese on top.

Nutrition

Calories: 97

Fat: 3.6 g

Carbs: 13.4g

Protein: 5 g

Beef Cabbage Stew

Preparation Time: 30 minutes

Cooking Time: 2 hours

Servings: 8

Ingredients

2 pounds beef stew meat

1 cube beef bouillon

8 ounce tomato sauce

¼ cup chopped celery

2 bay leaves

8 ounce plum tomatoes, chopped

1 1/3 cups hot chicken broth

Salt and pepper to taste

1 cabbage

1 tsp Greek seasoning

4 onions, chopped

Directions:

Cut off the stem of the cabbage. Separate the leaves carefully. Wash well and rinse off. Set aside for now.

In a large pan, fry the beef over medium low heat for about 8 to 10 minutes or until you get a brown color.

Into the pan, pour in 1/3 of the chicken broth.

Add the beef bouillon, and mix well.

Add the black pepper, salt and mix again.

Add the lid and cook on medium low heat for about 1 hour.

Take off the heat and transfer the mix into a bowl.

Spread the cabbage leaves on a flat surface.

Fill the middle using the beef mixture. Use generous portion of filling, it will give your stew a better taste.

Wrap the cabbage leaves tightly. Use a kitchen thread to tie it. Finish it with the remaining leaves and filling.

In a pot heat the oil over fry the onion for 1 minute.

Add the remaining chicken broth.

Add in the celery and tomato sauce and cook for another 10 minutes.

Add the Greek seasonings, and mix well. Bring to boil and then carefully add the wrapped cabbage.

Cover and cook for another 10 minutes.

Serve hot.

Nutrition

Calories: 372

Fat: 22.7 g

Carbs: 9g

Protein: 31.8 g

Quick Chili

Preparation Time: 10 minutes

Cooking Time: 1 hour

Servings: 4

Ingredients

½ pound lean ground beef

1 cup kidney beans

1 cup pumpkin, diced

2 cup water or stock

2 tablespoon hot pepper sauce

1 cup diced tomatoes

14 ounce tomato sauce

3 celery stalks, chopped

2 tablespoon oil

½ teaspoon chili powder

½ cup onion, chopped

6 ounce tomato paste

Directions

In a pressure cooker, add the oil and heat over medium heat.

Add the beef and fry until brown.

Transfer the beef into a plate and add the onion.

Fry until golden and then add the celery stalk, tomatoes and pumpkin.

Add the tomato paste, hot pepper sauce and cook for 5 minutes.

Add the bean and toss for 1 minute.

Add the beef and pour in the stock or water.

Cover with lid and cook on medium heat for 20 minutes.

Serve hot with rice or bread. Some even eat it as it is.

Nutrition

Calories: 248

Total Fat: 10g

Protein: 18g;

Total Carbs: 28.4g;

Fried Whole Tilapia

Preparation Time: 10 minutes

Cooking Time: 25 minutes

Servings: 2

Ingredients

10 ounce tilapia

2 tbsp oil

5 garlic cloves, mince

4 large onion, chopped

2 tbsp red chili powder

1 tsp turmeric powder

1 tsp cumin powder

1 tsp coriander powder

Salt to taste

Black pepper to taste

2 tbsp soy sauce

2 tbsp fish sauce

Directions:

Take the tilapia fish and clean it well without taking off the skin. You need to fry it whole, so you have to be careful about cleaning the gut inside.

Cut few slits on the skin so the seasoning gets inside well.

Marinate the fish with fish sauce, soy sauce, red chili powder, cumin powder, turmeric powder, coriander powder, salt and pepper.

Coat half of the onions in the same mixture too.

Let them marinate for 1 hour.

In a skillet heat the oil. Fry the fish for 8 minutes on each side.

Transfer the fish into serving plate.

Fry the marinated onions until they become crispy.

Add the remaining raw onions on top and serve hot.

Nutrition

Calories: 368

Fat: 30.1 g

Carbs: 9.2g

Protein: 16.6 g

African Chicken Curry

Preparation Time: 10 minutes

Cooking Time: 30 minutes

Servings: 4

Ingredients

1 pound whole chicken

1/2 onion

1/2 cup coconut milk

1/2 bay leaf

1-1/2 teaspoon olive oil

1/2 cup peeled tomatoes

1 teaspoon curry powder

1/8 teaspoon salt

1/2 lemon, juiced

1 clove garlic

Directions

Keep the skin of the chicken.

Cut your chicken into 8 pieces. It looks good when you keep the size not too small or not too big.

Discard the skin of the onion and garlic and mince the garlic and dice the onion.

Cut the tomato wedges.

Now in a pot add the olive oil and heat over medium heat.

Add the garlic and fry until it becomes brown.

Add the diced onion and caramelize it.

Add the bay leaf, and chicken pieces.

Fry the chicken pieces until they are golden.

Add the curry powder, coconut milk and salt.

Cover and cook for 10 minutes on high heat.

Turn the heat to medium low and add the lemon juice.

Add the tomato wedges and the coconut milk.

Cook for another 10 minutes.

Serve hot with rice or tortilla.

Nutrition

Calories: 354

Total Fat: 10g

Protein: 18g;

Total Carbs: 17g;

Yummy Garlic Chicken Livers

Preparation Time: 10 minutes

Cooking Time: 30 minutes

Servings: 2

Ingredients

½ pound chicken liver

2 teaspoon lime juice

6 garlic cloves, mince

½ teaspoon salt

1 tbsp ginger garlic paste

1 cup diced onion

1 tbsp red chili powder

1 tsp cumin

1 tsp coriander powder

Black pepper to taste

1 cardamom

2 tomatoes

1 cinnamon stick

1 bay leaf

4 tablespoon olive oil

Directions

In a large pan, heat your oil over high heat.

Add the garlic and fry them golden brown.

Add onion and fry until they become caramelized.

Turn the heat to medium and add the bay leaf, cinnamon stick, cardamom and toss for 30 seconds.

Add the ginger garlic paste and 1 tbsp water. Adding water prevents burning.

Add the coriander powder, black pepper, salt, cumin, and red chili powder.

Cover and cook on low heat for 3 minutes.

Add the livers and cook on medium heat for 15 minutes.

Add the tomatoes and cook for another 5 minutes.

Check the seasoning, add more salt if needed.

Serve hot with tortilla.

Nutrition

Calories: 174

Total Fat: 9g

Protein: 18g;

Total Carbs: 2.4g

Healthy Chickpea Burger

Preparation Time: 15 minutes

Cooking Time: 10 minutes

Servings: 2

Ingredients:

1 cup chickpeas, boiled

1 tbsp tomato puree

1 tsp soy sauce

A pinch of paprika

A pinch of white pepper

1 onion, diced

Salt to taste

2 lettuce leaves

½ cup bell pepper, sliced

1 tsp olive oil

1 avocado, sliced

2 Burger buns to serve

Directions:

Mash the chickpeas and combine with bell pepper, salt, pepper, paprika, soy sauce and tomato puree.

Use your hands to make patties.

Fry the patties golden brown with oil.

Assemble the burgers with lettuce, onion, avocado and enjoy.

Nutrition

Calories: 254

Total Fat: 12g

Protein: 9g;

Total Carbs: 7.8g;

Croutons Cabbage and Egg Salad

Preparation Time: 15 minutes

Cooking Time: 0 minutes

Servings: 2

Ingredients:

2 eggs, boiled

6-8 croutons

1 cup cabbage, cubed

½ cup lettuce, torn

2 tbsp cheddar cheese

½ cup Greek Yogurt

Salt to taste

White pepper to taste

Any nuts of your choice, chopped

Directions:

Cut the eggs into pieces.

Combine the yogurt, pepper, cheddar cheese, in a bowl.

Add the eggs, croutons, cabbage, lettuce, and nuts.

Serve.

Nutrition

Calories: 264

Total Fat: 14g

Protein: 14g;

Total Carbs: 8g;

Creamy Chicken Soup

Preparation Time: 15 minutes

Cooking Time: 30 minutes

Servings: 4

Ingredients:

1 egg, beaten

1 cup chicken breast, diced

1 tsp butter

1 tsp white pepper

1 cup milk

Salt to taste

1 cube of chicken stock

Fresh coriander

1 green chili

1 sprig of lemongrass

1 tsp lemon juice

Directions:

In a pressure cooker, add everything together and mix well.

Cover and cook on low heat for 10 minutes.

Stir once and again cook on medium high heat for 10 minutes.

Serve hot.

Nutrition

Calories: 364

Total Fat: 14g

Protein: 19g;

Total Carbs: 11g;

Chapter 13

Tips and Tricks for Women Over 50

Intermittent fasting is not easy. We need all the support and everything that can facilitate your trip. Here are some tricks that will facilitate your trip.

Decide your quick window.

Intermittent fasting is not a strict time-based diet. This means that you can choose the number of hours to fast and when to fast day or night. The periods of fasting and feeding are not essential to be the same every day.

Make sure you get enough sleep

When you get enough sleep, you become healthier, and your overall well-being is guaranteed. When we sleep, the body performs certain functions in the body that help burn calories and improve metabolic rate.

Eat healthily

Avoid eating what you want after a fast. Healthy meals should be the center of attention. They will help you get the necessary nutrients, such as vitamins, that will give you more energy during the fasting period.

Drink more water.

One of the best decisions you can make during a fast is to drink water. It will keep the body hydrated and drinking water before meals can significantly reduce appetite.

Start with something small.

If you have never tried it before, there is no way to start fasting and spend 48 hours without eating. To start, you can start eating at 20:00, for example, and you will have nothing left until 8 the next day. It will be easier because the dream is integrated into your window to eat.

Avoid stress Flickering can be difficult to do if you are stressed. This is because stress can trigger excessive food indulgence for some people. It is also easier to feed on garbage when stressed to feel better. That is why in intermittent fasting, it is recommended to avoid, if not control, stress levels. Be disciplined Remember that fasting means withdrawing food for a while. When fasting, be true to yourself and avoid eating before the appointed time. It will ensure that you lose maximum weight and benefit from intermittent fasting in healthy terms. vii. Keep drinks flavored. The most flavored drink says they are low in sugar, but in reality, they are not. Flavored drinks contain artificial sweeteners, which will negatively affect health. They will also increase your appetite, which will cause you to overeat, and this will cause you to gain weight instead of losing.

Find something to do when you fast. It is said that an inactive mind is the devil's workshop. When you fast intermittently and are not busy, you will think about food, and this will prevent you from fasting before the set time. You can run errands, listen to music, or even take a walk in the park.

You can train while fasting, but it is not mandatory. Mild exercises can also be done at home. When you train, you will develop muscle strength, and body fat will burn faster.

Differences between young and old.

At the most basic level, it should be said that there are detailed body differences between young women and older women. Many of these bodily differences are manifested by the external physical effects of aging, but many also occur within, far from what our eyes can see. As women age, enter, and leave menopause and mature fully, their bodies change, reflecting different nutritional needs for the next 30 years. During menopause, in particular, some foods help with impulses, hot flashes, and more, but the period of intense transition is more a door to a completely altered future (mental, physical, nutritional, and more). Women of this age experience a slower metabolism (with great frustration) and a decrease in hormone production. For weight and mood, therefore, menopause and maturation are equal disasters. Your body will become completely "out of control" compared to how it works. You are likely to gain weight despite the dietary choices you make, and you may feel that there is no relief in sight. Don't be fooled, however! Things may have changed for you, but they won't be stagnant changes. Basically, women in menopause and beyond need to absorb less energy in general from their food, but they need more protein to cope with the effects of aging. It will be necessary to increase vitamins B12 and D, calcium, and zinc, while the iron becomes less important for the aging of the female body. Vitamins C, E, A, and beta-carotene should also be increased to fight cancer, infections, diseases, and more. As women get older and mature even more, more things will change; mainly, it is no longer possible to give up these important supplements. In older and more mature women, the body's ability to recognize hunger and thirst is silenced, and dehydration represents a serious threat. Fewer calories are needed even for the older and more mature woman, but she still needs to eat as many nutrients (if not more!) Than the young woman. It seems that a younger woman can eat (relatively) what she wants and not worry about taking vitamins or supplements, but it is undeniable that the older woman will need this nutritional help to ensure longevity. Health needs become more pressing for women at this age, since their bodies are less flexible and resistant to problems that may arise.

Conclusion

Thank you for making it through to the end of this book. After being exposed to so much knowledge about intermittent fasting, you aren't likely to be surprised by the fact that the American Heart Association recommends intermittent fasting for losing weight. Its effectiveness in helping women lose weight is backed by science as well as by the personal experiences of thousands of women.

Fasting has existed in religious traditions for millennia, and now anyone can harness its health benefits with intermittent fasting. You don't have to undergo nearly the level of physical and mental fatigue of traditional water fasts, but you still see the difference in your waistline and in how you feel.

The scientific credibility that intermittent fasting has is all thanks to the biological process of autophagy. Autophagy is your body's natural means of getting rid of toxins that pollute your system. Intermittent fasting is your means of triggering this vital process.

Intermittent fasting is your ticket into triggering autophagy because it is easy to sustain. Unlike other means of achieving autophagy, intermittent fasting doesn't ask that you go to the gym or change what you eat (although you should still these things to get the most out of the biological process). Start your intermittent fast today and you will see all the health benefits uncovered in this book for yourself.